EXERCISE AND WOMEN'S HEALTH

EXERCISE AND WOMEN'S HEALTH

LAURA A. CHARLINGTON
EDITOR

Nova Science Publishers, Inc.
New York

For permission to use material from this book please contact us:
Telephone 631-231-7269; Fax 631-231-8175
Web Site: http://www.novapublishers.com

LIBRARY OF CONGRESS CATALOGING-IN-PUBLICATION DATA

Exercise and women's health / Laura A. Charlington (editor).
p. ; cm.
Includes bibliographical references and index.
ISBN 978-1-60456-013-8
1. Exercise--Physiological aspects. 2. Exercise--Health aspects. 3. Women--Health and hygiene. I. Charlington, Laura A.
[DNLM: 1. Exercise--physiology. 2. Exercise--psychology. 3. Women's Health. QT 255 E9554 2007]
QP301.E939 2007
613.7'1082--dc22

2007036482

Published by Nova Science Publishers, Inc. ✦ New York

CONTENTS

PREFACE

In the last 50 years significant numbers of men and women take little exercise in the course of their occupation. The computer keyboard, the rise of private transport, the world by television, household "labor saving" devices mean that with the minimal of physical effort people work and play. The benefits of doing regular exercise include a reduced risk of: heart disease, stroke, bowel cancer, breast cancer, osteoporosis, and obesity. In addition, many people feel better in themselves during and after exercise. Regular exercise is also thought to help ease stress, anxiety, and mild depression. This new book focuses on exercise and women's health.

Expert Commentary A - Loading is vital to the skeleton. Without loading the skeleton cannot attain adequate strength and is thus deemed to remain slender and fragile. Physical loading arising from different sports activities is associated not only with increased bone mass but also with robust bone structure. Bone structure is the key determinant of bone's ability to withstand the habitual loading without breaking over the life time. Particularly beneficial to bones seems to be loadings that involve high impacts. It is also obvious that young growing bones are more sensitive to exercise than adult bones.

Although physical activity induced effects on skeleton are evident, the skeleton's ability to preserve these benefits after the cessation of training is not clear. The effects can be expected to be lost if the osteogenic training was started in adulthood and the training is discontinued. In contrast, the exercise-induced bone gains obtained during the axial growth generally result in such a bone structure that largely keeps its rigidity despite the cessation of specific training. Obviously, at least moderate level of regular physical activity needs to be maintained

However, there still are many open questions in this topic. As regards the methodology, the most common bone trait in bone research is the areal BMD (mass over projected scan area) measured with dual-energy X-ray absorptiometry (DXA). Although precise and clinically feasible, DXA does not capture reliable information on whether the change in BMD is due to change in trabecular or cortical bone, or in combination – not to speak about structural details. Neither is it possible to reliably know whether the observed differences in BMD are attributable to bone size. DXA results are also subject to inaccuracies arising from differences in soft tissues. Altogether, DXA provides a severely suboptimal method to study the exercise effects on bone structure, and accordingly, the reliable information on bone structure has remained yet quite limited.

It is known that high-impact and odd-impact loadings are beneficial to bone, while repetitive low-impact loading is less effective. Nevertheless, there are still many imponderable questions regarding the specific amount, magnitude, and type of loading needed for getting anticipated osteogenic effects in different target groups. The number and intensity of impacts are not the only factors modulating the osteogenicity of exercise. Physical training may be more osteogenic if sufficient recovery periods are incorporated to the exercise regimes. Finally, convincing evidence on the dose-response relationships between specific exercises and effects on human bone structure wait for being revealed, although some preliminary results have been reported.

Expert Commentary B - Although usually misdiagnosed and ignored in the literature, exercise induced vasculitis (EIV, also described as exercise induced purpura and golfer's vasculitis) is a not uncommon skin disorder, occurring mostly in females after long walks, especially with hot weather.

Erythematous, urticarial or purpuric plaques arise on the lower legs, not involving skin compressed by socks, disappearing spontaneously after a few days, with frequent relapses at further muscular exercise. Symptoms include itch, pain, and burning sensation. Histopathology demonstrates leucocytoclastic vasculitis (or urticarial vasculitis). EIV is strictly cutaneous and does not involve other organs.

Short Communication - Iron is a nutritionally essential trace element that functions through incorporation into proteins and enzymes. Many of these proteins and enzymes, including hemoglobin, myoglobin, and cytochrome c, are essential for energy metabolism and physical performance. Iron deficiency affects a significant number of premenopausal women, due mainly to the combination of low dietary intake and iron losses through menstruation. It has been reported that the prevalence of iron deficiency is especially high in female athletes. Iron deficiency is associated with a series of negative consequences, including fatigue, diminished maximal work capacity, impaired aerobic adaptation, and reduced energetic efficiency. This chapter will focus on the effects of diminished iron status on performance in the female athlete. Potential causes of iron deficiency, including diet, impaired iron absorption, and increased whole body turnover will be addressed. Furthermore, the potential benefit of iron supplementation for certain female athletes will be discussed, to include a review of the available literature regarding iron supplementation and physical performance.

Chapter 1 - This chapter examines the perceptions of, and attitudes towards physical activity in older women, focusing upon the findings of structured face to face interviews conducted with a small sample of older Australian women. The women also completed an 'attitudes to physical activity questionnaire' and a one week activity diary. The data were analysed using content analysis techniques. The older women held various interpretations of the term 'physical activity' and these interpretations influenced their attitudes towards physical activity and actual reported behaviour. These perceptions need to be borne in mind when promoting physical activity amongst older women, when assessing older womens' readiness to become physically active and in interpreting their responses to questions about physical activity behaviour patterns. The findings are discussed within the context of the international evidence base, highlighting the public health implications for practitioners, policy makers and researchers.

Chapter 2 - The elderly represent a steadily growing proportion of the populations of the industrialized countries. This is particularly true for elderly women and the elderly over 80.

The physiological decline in the function of systems and apparatuses, the high prevalence of polipathology and the consequent increase in frailty and disability seen in the elderly imply increasing health-care and social burdens. The improvement in treatment of many pathologies affecting adults and older adults has brought about consistent increase in life expectancy and survival rates in these age groups. Nonetheless, maintenance of functional performance should be addressed more intensively, especially through life-style interventions and in particular through the implementation of physical activity programmes. Elderly women have a longer life expectancy and are at the same time more susceptible to frailty and functional decline. Thus they should be the main target of such an intervention. Unfortunately strong evidence in this subgroup is still lacking.

The objective of this review is to summarize the evidence about the effects of physical activity and physical exercise on total mortality, cardiovascular risk, obesity, diabetes, chronic diseases, cognitive and functional impairment, disability and quality of life in old women. In order to do so we analyzed meta-analyses, randomized-controlled trials (RCTs), longitudinal studies and non systematic reviews. A total of 18 studies matched our search criteria (2 meta-analyses, 4 RCTs, 8 longitudinal trials and 4 reviews).

Most of the analyzed studies showed that physical activity and exercise can improve the above-mentioned outcomes in samples of elderly women. The most acknowleged and consistent benefits of physical activity in older women are a longer life expectancy, a decrease, or at least a stabilization, in body weight, a lower incidence of diabetes complications and a lower incidence of functional impairment among the subjects affected by chronic diseases. Also quality of life is improved by physical activity according to most of the considered studies. In conclusion, physical activity can improve health condition and promote functional integrity in elderly women and thus physical activity appears to play a crucial role in the prevention and treatment of geriatric diseases. According to the evidence here revised, physical activity programmes should be implemented not only in the adults but even in the subgroup of elderly women, through educational campaigns or more individualized interventions.

Chapter 3 - Background and objectives: Physical exercise interventions are commonly used in the workplace to promote employees' physical and psychosocial functioning and work ability. However, there is limited scientific evidence of the effectiveness of such programmes, especially by gender. Also facts of dose-response effects on functioning or work ability are not yet fully understood. The aim of this study was to investigate among women office workers the effects of workplace physical exercise intervention on physical and psychosocial functioning, work ability, and general subjective well-being. Study is subgroup analyze of larger workplace intervention study.

Methods: 66 volunteer women [mean age 45.4 (SD 8.6) years] employees from four municipal administrative departments of Finland took part in a 15 weeks' cluster randomised cross-over design intervention. The intervention period consisted of light resistance training [30% 1RM (repetition maximum)] with guidance. The no-intervention period did not include any training or guidance. During the first five-week training period the training frequency was once in each working day, and thereafter 7-8 times a week. Musculoskeletal symptoms were measured using the Borg CR10 scales and muscular strength with a 5RM test. Psychosocial functioning, work ability and well-being variables were assessed by descriptive visual rating scales (0-100). Physical activity during the intervention was monitored by a weekly diary (training sessions and training time in minutes). Physical activity outside the intervention was recorded by the one-month all-time recall questionnaire (work, commuting, leisure time and miscellaneous time). The type of activity, frequency, duration and intensity of physical activity were converted to metabolic equivalent (MET) values. Statistical analyses were based on linear mixed models (SAS software). Subgroups analyses of women consisted of employees' who had restricted participation in daily activities because of musculoskeletal symptoms.

Results: Average training time was 122 minutes per 5-week (24 minutes/week, 5 minutes/working day). Load of training was average 342.0 MET minutes per 5-week. Compared with the non-intervention period the physical exercise intervention, resistance training and guidance together significantly decreased among subgroups of women employees' the intensity of headache [(p=0.004), mean difference 0.6 CR10, average percentual change 46%] and neck symptoms [(p=0.023), 0.3 CR10, 42%]. Whereas the active component of the intervention, light resistance training, resulted in significantly reduced intensity of symptoms in shoulder [(p=0.050), 0.27 CR10, 11%] and low back [(p=0.028), 0.45 CR10, 27%] symptoms. The light resistant training improved subjective physical well-being [(p=0.016), 5 units, 7%], physical condition [(p= 0.003), 6 units, 11%] and working ability [(p=0.045), 3 units, 3%,], but it did not affect the other psychosocial functioning and general well-being variables.

Conclusion: A physical exercise intervention, which included daily light resistance training, conducted during the working day affected on functioning and work ability in a positive direction among women office workers. A better understanding of physical exercise intervention's dose-response effects among women employees' can be helpful in maintaining functioning and work ability and preventing impairment in sedentary occupations.

Chapter 4 - Multiple sclerosis (MS) is a common neurological disease that primarily affects adult Caucasian women. Pain is a frequently reported symptom associated with MS with prevalence estimates ranging from 29% to 90% of patients. The pain associated with MS can interfere with activities of daily living and result in disability, and might be a barrier for participation in physical activity. Accordingly, pain might serve as a partial explanation for the predominance of physical inactivity in persons with MS. This study involved an examination of the relationships between several aspects of pain and self-report and objective measures of physical activity in two independent samples of women with MS (*N*s = 88 and 28). The women in both samples completed the Short-form of the McGill Pain Questionnaire (SF-MPQ) and then wore an accelerometer for seven days and completed the Godin Leisure-Time Exercise Questionnaire (GLTEQ). The SF-MPQ consists of 15 descriptors that yield sensory (SF-MPQS; sensory quality of pain), affective (SF-MPQA; affective qualities of pain), and overall or total (SF-MPQT) pain quality ratings. The SF-MPQ contains an additional item that measures the overall intensity of pain or Present Pain Index (PPI). We conducted Pearson product-moment correlations for examining the relationships between scores on the SF-MPQ, accelerometer, and GLTEQ in the two independent samples separately. Within the first sample ($N = 88$), there were significant correlations between the SF-MPQT ($r = -.29, p = .01$), SF-MPQS ($r = -.22, p = .04$), SF-MPQA ($r = -.39, p = .001$), and PPI ($r = -.29, p = .01$) scores and accelerometer counts. Scores from the SF-MPQ were not significantly correlated ($p > .05$) with GLTEQ scores. Within the second sample ($N = 28$), there was a similar pattern of results such that SF-MPQT ($r = -.40, p = .02$), SF-MPQS ($r = -.40, p = .02$), SF-MPQA ($r = -.30, p = .05$), and PPI ($r = -.45, p = .01$) scores from the SF-MPQ were significantly correlated with accelerometer counts. Again, scores from the SF-

MPQ were not significantly correlated ($p > .05$) with GLTEQ scores. The observed pattern of results indicates that sensory and affective dimensions of pain as well as the overall intensity of pain are associated with objectively measured physical activity in the two independent samples of individuals with MS. One potential implication is that pain does play a role in physical activity participation, but the relationship is not immediately recognized by participants based on the lack of relationships with the self-report measurement of physical activity.

Chapter 5 - This chapter provides the results of a study that compared the perceived, desired, and actual body images of 20 female students at a relatively small, primarily undergraduate university. Ten females were enrolled in a Human Kinetics (HK) program while the other 10 females were enrolled in other programs (Non-HK). Perceived and desired body images were determined from self-reported responses to a body image questionnaire. This body image questionnaire featured two questions associated with nine silhouettes that ranged in size from emaciated to obese. Actual body image was determined from anthropometric measurements and the applicable calculations for somatotype using the Heath-Carter Somatotype Calculations procedures. Descriptive statistics including means ± standard deviation were calculated for each group (i.e., HK and Non-HK) and the groups' perceived, desired, and actual body images compared using Oneway Analyses of Variance (ANOVA). Although, there were no significant differences ($p = .105$) in the body image satisfaction/dissatisfaction experienced between the HK and Non-HK groups, a high percentage (i.e., 70%) of the female students desired a smaller body image than what she perceived for herself. The ability to accurately identify one's actual body image was also not significantly ($p = .151$) different between the two groups. In fact, few females (i.e., 20%) accurately identified their body image from the nine silhouettes presented on the questionnaire. Thus, it was concluded that even though the female HK students were expected to know more about their body, including how and why their body moves, as well as a greater level of comfort with their physical body and how it moves, no significant differences existed in the perceived, desired, and actual body images of these female students compared to other females enrolled in Non-HK programs at a relatively small, primarily undergraduate university.

Chapter 6 - The objective of this exploratory one-group pre-post test study was to evaluate the nature of psychological change in inward depressed psychiatric patients attending a multi-disciplinary treatment, including psychomotor therapy. Female depressed psychiatric patients ($n = 51$) were examined before and after this program over a period of 3 months. The following psychological parameters were assessed by means of self-reporting questionnaires: depression, anxiety, global self-esteem, and physical self-worth. Patients demonstrated statistically significant improvements in depression, anxiety, global self-esteem and physical self-worth ($t(50)$ ranging from -3.76 to 4.65, all $p < 0.007$; ES ranging from 0.53 to -0.65). Changes in depression and anxiety displayed a strong negative correlation with changes in global self-esteem and physical self-worth (r varying from -0.39 to -0.67). Patients with greater improvement in physical self-worth reported greater improvement in anxiety and global self-esteem then patients who did not improve physical self-worth. Consequently, within the limitations of the research design it can be concluded that the program appeared successful in improving psychological well-being in female depressed patients. Results also provide preliminary insight into the potential role of physical self-worth in the recovery process of depressed patients.

Chapter 7 - This chapter discusses research regarding the area of physical activity, self-related health and the prevalence of overweight and body complaints in young women. The chapter integrates the results of a newly published Swedish investigation, and unpublished data from Norwegian and Australian studies regarding these topics.

It is generally accepted that physical activity provides benefits to health, functional ability and general quality of life. Physical activity also facilitates the development of motor skills and increases energy expenditure. Conversely, physical inactivity is a major public health challenge in the developed world and is recognized as a global epidemic. Furthermore, physical inactivity has emerged as an important risk factor for many chronic diseases as it has been shown to be closely related to an increased risk of cardiovascular disease, diabetes mellitus, osteoporosis and certain types of cancer. Therefore, participation in regular physical activity is important for improved bodily function and development. Unfortunately, levels of physical activity declines as young people mature, particularly among young women. European boys of all ages participate in more physical activity than European girls and the gender difference is more marked when vigorous activity is considered.

The most common argument is that young people's lack of participation in sport and physical activity is directly equated with a dramatic rise in childhood obesity. Accumulated evidence suggests that overweight youths become overweight adults, and inactive youths also become inactive adults.

Musculoskeletal symptoms are present early in school-age and it has been suggested that these early symptoms might represent the start of a lifelong course of musculoskeletal complaints. The prevalence of the various definitions of low back pain increased greatly in the early teen years, earlier for girls than for boys. By the ages of 18 years for girls and 20 years for boys, more than 50 % had experienced at least one low back pain episode. There is a general tendency for more young women to report low back pain than young men.

Previous studies have shown that walking and cycling to school are associated with higher physical activity levels therefore correlating that active travel to school provides an opportunity for daily physical activity. Furthermore, schools should provide opportunities for young women to participate in a wider range of activities such as dancing, gymnastics, aerobics etc. to increase their physical activity and improve their health.

Chapter 8 - The purpose of this chapter is to present an overview of evidence on the effects of exercise in women living with HIV in order to identify directions for future research. To this end, the authors present a synthesis of research on a variety of HIV and exercise outcomes, including immunological, virological, cardiopulmonary, musculoskeletal, body composition and psychological effects, with reflection on the relevance of these findings for women. The authors conclude that, given (a) the significance of exercise as a therapeutic strategy for people living with HIV, (b) the feminization of the HIV pandemic, (c) the unique considerations related to gender and exercise, and (d) the paucity of evidence on the effects of exercise in women living with HIV, further research is urgently needed to explore the safety and effectiveness of aerobic and progressive resistive exercise in women living with HIV. Such research should take into account methodological lessons learned from existing studies, which have been conducted primarily with male adults living with HIV. Future research should also take into account unique considerations pertaining to women living with HIV, including metabolic and hormonal features, as well as the different social demands, circumstances and context of women's lives.

In: Exercise and Women's Health
Editor: Laura A. Charlington, pp. 1-9
ISBN: 978-1-60456-013-8

Expert Commentary A

COMMENTARY ON PHYSICAL ACTIVITY AND BONE HEALTH

Kirsti Uusi-Rasi and Harri Sievänen
The UKK Institute for Health Promotion Research, Tampere, Finland

ABSTRACT

Loading is vital to the skeleton. Without loading the skeleton cannot attain adequate strength and is thus deemed to remain slender and fragile. Physical loading arising from different sports activities is associated not only with increased bone mass but also with robust bone structure. Bone structure is the key determinant of bone's ability to withstand the habitual loading without breaking over the life time. Particularly beneficial to bones seems to be loadings that involve high impacts. It is also obvious that young growing bones are more sensitive to exercise than adult bones.

Although physical activity induced effects on skeleton are evident, the skeleton's ability to preserve these benefits after the cessation of training is not clear. The effects can be expected to be lost if the osteogenic training was started in adulthood and the training is discontinued. In contrast, the exercise-induced bone gains obtained during the axial growth generally result in such a bone structure that largely keeps its rigidity despite the cessation of specific training. Obviously, at least moderate level of regular physical activity needs to be maintained

However, there still are many open questions in this topic. As regards the methodology, the most common bone trait in bone research is the areal BMD (mass over projected scan area) measured with dual-energy X-ray absorptiometry (DXA). Although precise and clinically feasible, DXA does not capture reliable information on whether the change in BMD is due to change in trabecular or cortical bone, or in combination – not to speak about structural details. Neither is it possible to reliably know whether the observed differences in BMD are attributable to bone size. DXA results are also subject to inaccuracies arising from differences in soft tissues. Altogether, DXA provides a severely suboptimal method to study the exercise effects on bone structure, and accordingly, the reliable information on bone structure has remained yet quite limited.

It is known that high-impact and odd-impact loadings are beneficial to bone, while repetitive low-impact loading is less effective. Nevertheless, there are still many imponderable questions regarding the specific amount, magnitude, and type of loading needed for getting anticipated osteogenic effects in different target groups. The number and intensity of impacts are not the only factors modulating the osteogenicity of exercise. Physical training may be more osteogenic if sufficient recovery periods are incorporated to the exercise regimes. Finally, convincing evidence on the dose-response relationships between specific exercises and effects on human bone structure wait for being revealed, although some preliminary results have been reported.

BONE MASS AND STRUCTURE

The skeleton can be considered as having a multifaceted role. The flat bones, such as the ribs and those of the skull, protect the vital organs they surround. The long bones provide rigid lever arms for muscles to pull against, while being as light as possible to allow efficient locomotion. Bone adaptation during skeletal growth and development continuously adjusts skeletal mass and shape to changing mechanical environments [1, 2]. Bone strength is not a direct consequence of bone mass, but in particular, the consequence of cortical and trabecular bone structure, geometry and microarchitecture. In other words, it is crucial how the bone mass is spatially distributed. Naturally, proper material properties of bone are a prerequisite for bone strength [3, 4].

Physical activity plays an important role not only on the process of bone modeling and remodeling but also in shaping a mechanically appropriate bone structure [1, 2]. Ignoring the evident geometrical adaptation of bone to loading can lead to underestimation of the influence of loading on bone strength in general, and interfere the assessment of specific effects of different loading types on skeleton. Although the exact type of loading that would optimally improve bone strength is not yet established, there is strong experimental and clinical evidence that impact loading (skeletal loading consisting of highly accelerating and decelerating movements, especially from non-habitual directions), produces sufficiently high loading magnitudes and rates exceeding the threshold level required for osteogenic stimulus [5-11].

Apparently, the capacity of the human skeleton to adapt to physical training is substantially different between childhood and adulthood. Exercise at childhood stimulates the bone modelling process, expanding bone size to produce a larger and robust bone. The effect of exercise on bone size, particularly on the long bone epiphyseal sites, is generally less effective once axial growth has ceased. Training started before or at puberty seems to be more effective for high accrual of bone mass and consequent strengthening of bone [12-18]. For growing skeleton, the most effective training type seem to be sports that involve jumps, leaps, high impacts, and high accelerations or deceleration movements through intense exercises. Also odd impacts or dynamic loading from atypical directions are effective [8].

After rapid bone mineral accumulation in late adolescence, peak bone mass is though to be attained around the age 20 [19, 20]. However, the peak in BMD does not necessarily mean peak in bone strength, as shown in a longitudinal study of Petit et al. [21]. There may be age-related differences in the way bone responds to mechanical loading, but sensitivity to mechanical loading does not end with completion of the juvenile growth period. Relatively slow but cumulative changes in bone mass and structure occur in adults, especially among younger adults [2]. Healthy premenopausal women may reach effective impact intensities through normal physical training activities. High-impact and exceptional strain-producing loading regimens, such as jumping or resistance training, has been shown to be effective on strengthening of bones [6, 11, 22]. Even though the changes in bone geometry and strength indices observed during the 12-mo intervention are generally relatively small (0.5 – 2.0%) [23-28], if continued for several years, the cumulative influence on bone strength may become relevant.

While exercise-induced effects on bones apparently decline with age, there still is a possibility of a significant adaptation to loading in older age. Meta-analysis based on intervention studies including different type of training, such as brisk walking, jogging, rowing, stair climbing or jumping exercise, affirm that physical activity may prevent bone loss, and even slightly improve bone mass among postmenopausal women [23, 28-30]. Even though the direct training effect on bone mass or structure may be limited, exercise can be effective method to prevent falls in improving many of the risk factors of falling, such as gait, balance, coordination, reaction time and muscle strength. Several studies suggest that high-impact loading, such as jumping, strength-training, or a combination of resistance and jumping training can maintain, or even slightly increase bone mass in postmenopausal and elderly women [31-36]. In fact, the loss of muscle strength and power as well as aerobic capacity may lead to further decrease in activity, and an inability to continue such activities that provide an adequate stimulus to maintain bone mass.

In addition to maintenance of bone mass, exercise can reshape the bone structure and geometry by improving the cortical bone properties, e.g. cortical thickness. A classic example of this is the study by Adami et al. [37], which besides showing specific training effects on bone pinpointed the importance of structural evaluation of bones with appropriate methods. Adami and co-workers found no significant training effect with conventional DXA-based BMD-measurements, while the cortical area increased at apparent expense of the trabecular bone in response to loading. Exercise may change the bone mass distribution, and for example, the change in trabecular-to-cortical bone ratio may play an important role in determining bone strength, since changes in cortical bone are essential in improving bone strength [38, 39].

However, one additional interesting question is, if the exercise-induced benefits are maintained after cessation of training. it has been suggested that structural changes obtained during the skeletal growth could be, at least, partially maintained even if exercise is decreased [40-42]. In adults, the exercise-induced improvements in physical performance, such as muscle power and agility, are more significant than improvements in bone mass, particularly when assessing the role of exercise in reducing the risk of fragility fractures. However, it is apparent that exercise-induced benefits will mainly be lost if exercise is completely ceased, and thus continued training is needed to maintain the positive effects of physical activity.

Measurement Methods

Concerning the findings of exercise effects on bone reviewed above, it is stressed again that it is more important to show an exercise effect on robustness of the bone than on its BMD.

The most common bone trait in bone research have been the areal BMD (mass over projected scan area) measured with dual-energy X-ray absorptiometry (DXA). Although precise and clinically feasible, DXA does not capture reliable information on whether the change in BMD is due to change in trabecular or cortical bone, or in combination – not to speak about structural details. Neither is it possible to reliably know whether the observed differences in BMD are attributable to bone size. Besides the ambiguity in interpretation [43], DXA results are also subject to inaccuracies arising from differences in soft tissues [44].

Obviously the commonly used DXA provides a severely suboptimal method to study the exercise effects on bone structure, and accordingly, the reliable information on bone structure has remained yet quite limited. Instead, peripheral quantitative computed tomography (pQCT) provides a feasible method to study the exercise effects on coarse bone structure [45]. The pQCT method have been used only in a few exercise interventions [36-38, 46] but much more in cross-sectional studies of athletes [9, 47-49]. It is recalled that the pQCT-measured density values reflect only the apparent density of trabecular tissue and cortical bone, being thus lumped measures of the scanned bone volume without any structural details. For this reason, the observed change in cortical volumetric density can be interpreted as changed general porosity of cortical bone. The change in the trabecular bone can be interpreted as thinning/thickening and perforation/increased connectivity within the trabecular structure. In this respect, the possibility to assess trabecular structure in detail by high-resolution 3-D pQCT is interesting and promising [50]. Also magnetic resonance imaging may offer a reasonable tool to study bone structures without radiation dose [51].

Dose-Response

In the pharmacological treatment the concept of dosage is vital. Physicians normally start with a dose of a drug believed to be the minimum effective dose, and this initial dose may then be titrated upwards if no response to treatment is seen in the given patient. Some analogy between physical activity and drugs can be brought up; exercise causes many physiological changes in the body, and helps to prevent the development of many chronic diseases. It is plausible that there is a minimum dose of physical activity for health benefits, that these benefits increase with increasing dose, and that beyond a certain dose, adverse effects outweigh benefits [52]. Mechanical loading influences on bone mass and architecture most probably through the dynamic strains it engenders into bone tissue. Peak strain amplitude and strain rate are determinants of osteogenic response. There is also a threshold, which must be surpassed before osteogenic stimulus is initiated.[53]

It is established that physical activity can help to maintain bone mass [28, 29] and with high probability also to prevent fragility fractures [54-56] , there is not yet a consensus about the quality and quantity of exercise needed for effective results. It is not easy to define the minimum effective dose, when exercise is used as treatment, and on the other hand, the maximum dose still known to be safe. Cross-sectional studies of athletes provide a convenient means to study the extremes, particularly the ultimate potential of specific exercise to increase bone robustness – feasible exercise doses should be found at lower levels. The dose-response may also depend on age, sex, medication, or ethnic/racial differences [57, 58]. It may even be that the female skeleton is more responsive to mechanical loading after menopause than during fertile years. Young women have higher bone mass than young men, probably due to an estrogen-driven packing of extra mineral into female bones around puberty and an unpacking at menopause [59]. Apparently the individual responses show substantial variation to exercise that can complicate setting the exercise dose.

Despite many open questions, some guidelines can be given. Skeletal adaptation to loading is evidently affected by the magnitude of the strains within the bones, the strain rate, the strain distribution, and the number and frequency of repetitions. It has been shown that osteogenic threshold level required to increase bone mass is achieved at accelerations higher than 3.9 g, which approximate to jumping or running [11]. It is good to note that low-impact exercise can initiate redistribution of bone mass, while higher threshold is needed to increase bone mass [46]. Even though high-impact loading is effective among young healthy women, it may not be so for all, and especially not for older people, e.g. with fragile bones or other musculoskeltal troubles. On the other hand, regular jumping exercises have been found tentatively effective among elderly, including osteoporotic women, in reducing the number of fractures [60].

Walking or stair climbing may not be as effective on bone mass or density as previously mentioned jumping or running. It may be that these types of activity do not generate sufficient strain magnitudes and rates to produce bone accrual or at least maintenance of the existing bone structure. However, miles walked per day have been shown to be positively associated with bone size at the femoral neck. Because this is an important common fractures site, and because larger bones are generally stronger than smaller bones with equal quality, this apparent effect of walking on bone size may be important in reducing fracture risk, despite its apparent lack of effect on bone mass [58]. Walking activity is associated with reduced incidence of hip fractures [54].

Turner has summarized the principles of bone adaptation to mechanical stimuli: 1) bone adaptation is driven by dynamic, rather than static, loading; 2) only a short duration of mechanical loading is necessary to initiate adaptive response, while extending the loading has a diminishing effect on further adaptation; and 3) bone cells accommodate to customary loading environment, making them less responsive to routine loading stimuli. In addition to the number and intensity of impacts, the rest period between the loads increases the osteogenic response [61]. For example, bone looses more than 95% of its mechanosensitivity after only 20 loading cycles. A 4-hour rest period between the loading bouts will double the loading induced bone formation, and after 24-hour rest 98% of the bone mechanosensitivity will be returned [62]. These simple principles are still valid as to the current understanding of skeletal responsiveness to physical loading and exercise.

Future clinical intervention trials investigating the effects of exercise on fragility fractures and their risk factors should be based on (1) reliable assessments of whole-bone structure; (2) measurements of exercise-induced loading, muscle performance, and balance in real-life situations; and (3) collection of data on falls and fractures [56].

References

[1] Frost, H.M. (2003) Bone's mechanostat: a 2003 update. *Anat. Rec. A Discov. Mol. Cell Evol. Biol*, *275*, 1081-1101.

[2] Ruff, C., Holt, B. & Trinkaus, E. (2006) Who's afraid of the big bad Wolff?: "Wolff's law" and bone functional adaptation. *Am. J. Phys. Anthropol*, *129*, 484-498.

[3] Jarvinen, T.L., Sievanen, H., Jokihaara, J. & Einhorn, T.A. (2005) Revival of bone strength: the bottom line. *J. Bone Miner Res*, *20*, 717-720.

[4] Sievanen, H., Kannus, P. & Jarvinen, T.L. (2007) Bone Quality: An Empty Term. *PloS. Med*, *4*, e27.

[5] Heinonen, A., Oja, P., Kannus, P., Sievanen, H., Haapasalo, H., Manttari, A. & Vuori, I. (1995) Bone mineral density in female athletes representing sports with different loading characteristics of the skeleton. *Bone*, *17*, 197-203.

[6] Heinonen, A., Kannus, P., Sievanen, H., Oja, P., Pasanen, M., Rinne, M., Uusi-Rasi, K. & Vuori, I. (1996) Randomised controlled trial of effect of high-impact exercise on selected risk factors for osteoporotic fractures. *Lancet*, *348*, 1343-1347.

[7] Helge, E.W. & Kanstrup, I.L. (2002) Bone density in female elite gymnasts: impact of muscle strength and sex hormones. *Med. Sci. Sports Exerc*, *34*, 174-180.

[8] Nikander, R., Sievanen, H., Heinonen, A. & Kannus, P. (2005) Femoral neck structure in adult female athletes subjected to different loading modalities. *J. Bone Miner Res*, *20*, 520-528.

[9] Nikander, R., Sievanen, H., Uusi-Rasi, K., Heinonen, A. & Kannus, P. (2006) Loading modalities and bone structures at nonweight-bearing upper extremity and weight-bearing lower extremity: a pQCT study of adult female athletes. *Bone*, *39*, 886-894.

[10] Proctor, K.L., Adams, W.C., Shaffrath, J.D. & Van Loan, M.D. (2002) Upper-limb bone mineral density of female collegiate gymnasts versus controls. *Med. Sci. Sports Exerc*, *34*, 1830-1835.

[11] Vainionpaa, A., Korpelainen, R., Leppaluoto, J. & Jamsa, T. (2005) Effects of high-impact exercise on bone mineral density: a randomized controlled trial in premenopausal women. *Osteoporos Int*, *16*, 191-197.

[12] Kannus, P., Haapasalo, H., Sankelo, M., Sievanen, H., Pasanen, M., Heinonen, A., Oja, P. & Vuori, I. (1995) Effect of starting age of physical activity on bone mass in the dominant arm of tennis and squash players. *Ann. Intern. Med*, *123*, 27-31.

[13] Heinonen, A., Sievanen, H., Kannus, P., Oja, P., Pasanen, M. & Vuori, I. (2000) High-impact exercise and bones of growing girls: a 9-month controlled trial. *Osteoporos Int*, *11*, 1010-1017.

[14] Bradney, M., Pearce, G., Naughton, G., Sullivan, C., Bass, S., Beck, T., Carlson, J. & Seeman, E. (1998) Moderate exercise during growth in prepubertal boys: changes in bone mass, size, volumetric density, and bone strength: a controlled prospective study. *J. Bone Miner. Res*, *13*, 1814-1821.

[15] Bass, S., Pearce, G., Bradney, M., Hendrich, E., Delmas, P.D., Harding, A. & Seeman, E. (1998) Exercise before puberty may confer residual benefits in bone density in adulthood: studies in active prepubertal and retired female gymnasts. *J. Bone Miner Res*, *13*, 500-507.

[16] Morris, F.L., Naughton, G.A., Gibbs, J.L., Carlson, J.S. & Wark, J.D. (1997) Prospective ten-month exercise intervention in premenarcheal girls: positive effects on bone and lean mass. *J. Bone Miner Res*, *12*, 1453-1462.

[17] McKay, H.A., Petit, M.A., Schutz, R.W., Prior, J.C., Barr, S.I. & Khan, K.M. (2000) Augmented trochanteric bone mineral density after modified physical education classes: a randomized school-based exercise intervention study in prepubescent and early pubescent children. *J. Pediatr*, *136*, 156-162. rt&artType=abs&id=a102917&target=.

[18] Wang, Q.J., Suominen, H., Nicholson, P.H., Zou, L.C., Alen, M., Koistinen, A. & Cheng, S. (2005) Influence of physical activity and maturation status on bone mass and geometry in early pubertal girls. *Scand J. Med. Sci. Sports*, *15*, 100-106.

[19] Haapasalo, H., Kannus, P., Sievanen, H., Pasanen, M., Uusi-Rasi, K., Heinonen, A., Oja, P. & Vuori, I. (1996) Development of mass, density, and estimated mechanical characteristics of bones in Caucasian females. *J. Bone Miner Res*, *11*, 1751-1760.

[20] Matkovic, V., Jelic, T., Wardlaw, G.M., Ilich, J.Z., Goel, P.K., Wright, J.K., Andon, M.B., Smith, K.T. & Heaney, R.P. (1994) Timing of peak bone mass in Caucasian females and its implication for the prevention of osteoporosis. Inference from a cross-sectional model. *J. Clin. Invest*, *93*, 799-808.

[21] Petit, M.A., Beck, T.J., Lin, H.M., Bentley, C., Legro, R.S. & Lloyd, T. (2004) Femoral bone structural geometry adapts to mechanical loading and is influenced by sex steroids: the Penn State Young Women's Health Study. *Bone*, *35*, 750-759.

[22] Friedlander, A.L., Genant, H.K., Sadowsky, S., Byl, N.N. & Gluer, C.C. (1995) A two-year program of aerobics and weight training enhances bone mineral density of young women. *J. Bone Miner Res*, *10*, 574-585.

[23] Kelley, G.A. (1998) Exercise and regional bone mineral density in postmenopausal women: a meta-analytic review of randomized trials. *Am. J. Phys. Med. Rehabil*, *77*, 76-87.

[24] Kelley, G.A., Kelley, K.S. & Tran, Z.V. (2001) Resistance training and bone mineral density in women: a meta-analysis of controlled trials. *Am. J. Phys. Med. Rehabil*, *80*, 65-77.

[25] Kelley, G.A., Kelley, K.S. & Tran, Z.V. (2002) Exercise and lumbar spine bone mineral density in postmenopausal women: a meta-analysis of individual patient data. *J. Gerontol. A Biol. Sci. Med. Sci*, *57*, M599-604.

[26] Bonaiuti, D., Shea, B., Iovine, R., Negrini, S., Robinson, V., Kemper, H.C., Wells, G., Tugwell, P. & Cranney, A. (2002) Exercise for preventing and treating osteoporosis in postmenopausal women. *Cochrane Database Syst. Rev*, CD000333.

[27] Shea, B., Bonaiuti, D., Iovine, R., Negrini, S., Robinson, V., Kemper, H.C., Wells, G., Tugwell, P. & Cranney, A. (2004) Cochrane Review on exercise for preventing and treating osteoporosis in postmenopausal women. *Eura Medicophys*, *40*, 199-209.

[28] Wolff, I., van Croonenborg, J.J., Kemper, H.C., Kostense, P.J. & Twisk, J.W. (1999) The effect of exercise training programs on bone mass: a meta-analysis of published controlled trials in pre- and postmenopausal women. *Osteoporos Int*, *9*, 1-12.

[29] Wallace, B.A. & Cumming, R.G. (2000) Systematic review of randomized trials of the effect of exercise on bone mass in pre- and postmenopausal women. *Calcif. Tissue Int*, *67*, 10-18.

[30] Kelley, G. (1998) Aerobic exercise and lumbar spine bone mineral density in postmenopausal women: a meta-analysis. *J. Am. Geriatr. Soc*, *46*, 143-152.

[31] Pruitt, L.A., Taaffe, D.R. & Marcus, R. (1995) Effects of a one-year high-intensity versus low-intensity resistance training program on bone mineral density in older women. *J. Bone Miner Res*, *10*, 1788-1795.

[32] Kohrt, W.M., Snead, D.B., Slatopolsky, E. & Birge, S.J., Jr. (1995) Additive effects of weight-bearing exercise and estrogen on bone mineral density in older women. *J. Bone Miner Res*, *10*, 1303-1311.

[33] Kohrt, W.M., Ehsani, A.A. & Birge, S.J., Jr. (1997) Effects of exercise involving predominantly either joint-reaction or ground-reaction forces on bone mineral density in older women. *J. Bone Miner Res*, *12*, 1253-1261.

[34] Kerr, D., Ackland, T., Maslen, B., Morton, A. & Prince, R. (2001) Resistance training over 2 years increases bone mass in calcium-replete postmenopausal women. *J. Bone Miner Res*, *16*, 175-181.

[35] Liu-Ambrose, T.Y., Khan, K.M., Eng, J.J., Heinonen, A. & McKay, H.A. (2004) Both resistance and agility training increase cortical bone density in 75- to 85-year-old women with low bone mass: a 6-month randomized controlled trial. *J. Clin. Densitom*, *7*, 390-398.

[36] Karinkanta, S., Heinonen, A., Sievanen, H., Uusi-Rasi, K., Pasanen, M., Ojala, K., Fogelholm, M. & Kannus, P. (2007) A multi-component exercise regimen to prevent functional decline and bone fragility in home-dwelling elderly women: randomized, controlled trial. *Osteoporos Int*, *18*, 453-462.

[37] Adami, S., Gatti, D., Braga, V., Bianchini, D. & Rossini, M. (1999) Site-specific effects of strength training on bone structure and geometry of ultradistal radius in postmenopausal women. *J. Bone Miner Res*, *14*, 120-124.

[38] Uusi-Rasi, K., Kannus, P., Cheng, S., Sievanen, H., Pasanen, M., Heinonen, A., Nenonen, A., Halleen, J., Fuerst, T., Genant, H. & Vuori, I. (2003) Effect of alendronate and exercise on bone and physical performance of postmenopausal women: a randomized controlled trial. *Bone*, *33*, 132-143.

[39] Cheng, S., Sipila, S., Taaffe, D.R., Puolakka, J. & Suominen, H. (2002) Change in bone mass distribution induced by hormone replacement therapy and high-impact physical exercise in post-menopausal women. *Bone*, *31*, 126-135.

[40] Kontulainen, S., Kannus, P., Haapasalo, H., Heinonen, A., Sievanen, H., Oja, P. & Vuori, I. (1999) Changes in bone mineral content with decreased training in competitive young adult tennis players and controls: a prospective 4-yr follow-up. *Med. Sci. Sports Exerc*, *31*, 646-652.

[41] Kontulainen, S., Kannus, P., Haapasalo, H., Sievanen, H., Pasanen, M., Heinonen, A., Oja, P. & Vuori, I. (2001) Good maintenance of exercise-induced bone gain with decreased training of female tennis and squash players: a prospective 5-year follow-up study of young and old starters and controls. *J. Bone Miner Res*, *16*, 195-201.

[42] Nordstrom, A., Karlsson, C., Nyquist, F., Olsson, T., Nordstrom, P. & Karlsson, M. (2005) Bone loss and fracture risk after reduced physical activity. *J. Bone Miner Res*, *20*, 202-207.

[43] Sievanen, H. (2000) A physical model for dual-energy X-ray absorptiometry--derived bone mineral density. *Invest. Radiol*, *35*, 325-330.

[44] Bolotin, H.H. & Sievanen, H. (2001) Inaccuracies inherent in dual-energy X-ray absorptiometry in vivo bone mineral density can seriously mislead diagnostic/prognostic interpretations of patient-specific bone fragility. *J. Bone Miner Res*, *16*, 799-805.

[45] Sievanen, H., Koskue, V., Rauhio, A., Kannus, P., Heinonen, A. & Vuori, I. (1998) Peripheral quantitative computed tomography in human long bones: evaluation of in vitro and in vivo precision. *J. Bone Miner Res*, *13*, 871-882.

[46] Vainionpaa, A., Korpelainen, R., Sievanen, H., Vihriala, E., Leppaluoto, J. & Jamsa, T. (2007) Effect of impact exercise and its intensity on bone geometry at weight-bearing tibia and femur. *Bone*, *40*, 604-611.

[47] Kontulainen, S., Sievanen, H., Kannus, P., Pasanen, M. & Vuori, I. (2002) Effect of long-term impact-loading on mass, size, and estimated strength of humerus and radius of female racquet-sports players: a peripheral quantitative computed tomography study between young and old starters and controls. *J. Bone Miner Res*, *17*, 2281-2289.

[48] Liu, L., Maruno, R., Mashimo, T., Sanka, K., Higuchi, T., Hayashi, K., Shirasaki, Y., Mukai, N., Saitoh, S. & Tokuyama, K. (2003) Effects of physical training on cortical bone at midtibia assessed by peripheral QCT. *J. Appl. Physiol*, *95*, 219-224.

[49] Heinonen, A., Sievanen, H., Kyrolainen, H., Perttunen, J. & Kannus, P. (2001) Mineral mass, size, and estimated mechanical strength of triple jumpers' lower limb. *Bone*, *29*, 279-285.

[50] Khosla, S., Riggs, B.L., Atkinson, E.J., Oberg, A.L., McDaniel, L.J., Holets, M., Peterson, J.M. & Melton, L.J., 3rd. (2006) Effects of sex and age on bone microstructure at the ultradistal radius: a population-based noninvasive in vivo assessment. *J. Bone Miner Res*, *21*, 124-131.

[51] Sievanen, H., Karstila, T., Apuli, P. & Kannus, P. (2007) Magnetic resonance imaging of the femoral neck cortex. *Acta Radiol*, *48*, 308-314.

[52] Lee, I.M. (2007) Dose-response relation between physical activity and fitness: even a little is good; more is better. *Jama*, *297*, 2137-2139.

[53] Mosley, J.R., March, B.M., Lynch, J. & Lanyon, L.E. (1997) Strain magnitude related changes in whole bone architecture in growing rats. *Bone*, *20*, 191-198.

[54] Feskanich, D., Willett, W. & Colditz, G. (2002) Walking and leisure-time activity and risk of hip fracture in postmenopausal women. *Jama*, *288*, 2300-2306.

[55] Michaelsson, K., Olofsson, H., Jensevik, K., Larsson, S., Mallmin, H., Berglund, L., Vessby, B. & Melhus, H. (2007) Leisure Physical Activity and the Risk of Fracture in Men. *PLoS Med*, *4*, e199.

[56] Sievanen, H. & Kannus, P. (2007) Physical Activity Reduces the Risk of Fragility Fracture. *PLoS Med*, *4*, e222.

[57] Duan, Y., Beck, T.J., Wang, X.F. & Seeman, E. (2003) Structural and biomechanical basis of sexual dimorphism in femoral neck fragility has its origins in growth and aging. *J. Bone Miner Res*, *18*, 1766-1774.

[58] Havill, L.M., Mahaney, M.C., T, L.B. & Specker, B.L. (2007) Effects of genes, sex, age, and activity on BMC, bone size, and areal and volumetric BMD. *J. Bone Miner Res*, *22*, 737-746.

[59] Jarvinen, T.L., Kannus, P. & Sievanen, H. (2003) Estrogen and bone--a reproductive and locomotive perspective. *J. Bone Miner Res*, *18*, 1921-1931.

[60] Korpelainen, R., Keinanen-Kiukaanniemi, S., Heikkinen, J., Vaananen, K. & Korpelainen, J. (2006) Effect of exercise on extraskeletal risk factors for hip fractures in elderly women with low BMD: a population-based randomized controlled trial. *J. Bone Miner Res*, *21*, 772-779.

[61] Turner, C.H. (1998) Three rules for bone adaptation to mechanical stimuli. *Bone*, *23*, 399-407.

[62] Turner, C.H. & Robling, A.G. (2005) Exercises for improving bone strength. *Br. J. Sports Med*, *39*, 188-189.

In: Exercise and Women's Health
Editor: Laura A. Charlington, pp. 11-16

ISBN: 978-1-60456-013-8

Expert Commentary B

EXERCISE INDUCED VASCULITIS

Albert-Adrien Ramelet[*]

ABSTRACT

Although usually misdiagnosed and ignored in the literature, exercise induced vasculitis (EIV, also described as exercise induced purpura and golfer's vasculitis) is a not uncommon skin disorder, occurring mostly in females after long walks, especially with hot weather.

Erythematous, urticarial or purpuric plaques arise on the lower legs, not involving skin compressed by socks, disappearing spontaneously after a few days, with frequent relapses at further muscular exercise. Symptoms include itch, pain, and burning sensation. Histopathology demonstrates leucocytoclastic vasculitis (or urticarial vasculitis). EIV is strictly cutaneous and does not involve other organs.

Key words: Purpura; vasculitis; exercise; marathon; long distance runners; walking; hiking; golf.

DEFINITION

Exercise induced vasculitis (EIV) is a strictly cutaneous affection, consisting in an erythematous, urticarial, or purpuric itchy eruption on the lower legs of healthy patients, occurring especially after a long walk in hot weather, spontaneously disappearing after some days, relapsing after similar exercises, with a leucoclastic or urticarial vasculitis at the histopathology.

[*] Correspondance to: Dr Albert-Adrien Ramelet; 2 place Benjamin Constant; CH-1003 Lausanne (Switzerland); aar@ramelet-dr.ch

Epidemiology

Prevalence of EIV is unknown. EIV occurs at the legs after a sustained exercise, as walking or hiking, especially after mountain climbing, or if walking when wearing unsuitable shoes [1-6]. Hot climate is a prerequisite, although milder eruptions may also occur in some patients at a colder season. Sun exposure does not appear as a contributory factor [1-9].

Skin specialists seldom observe such patients, as the condition fades within a few days and occurs during leisure.

The disorder is certainly not uncommon. Since our original description of EIV [1-6], we observed or received by mail numerous new cases of EIV, mostly in women suffering from lipedema. In our experience, EIV is unusual in male hikers. However it has been observed in several male golfers [10]. In the special form of EIV occurring after effort close to exhaustion, 54 male and female announced themselves spontaneously to a medical investigators' team at the end of a night 80 km race [7-9].

Few publications have been devoted to EIV. In most published series [1-6.11-12], there is a clear female preponderance, which may be explained by the association of the disorder, with lipedema. Family cases have been reported [3].

Physiopathology

The aetiology of EIV is still unknown. Two hypotheses are worth noting, failure of thermoregulation, and decrease of venous drainage [2,3,7,8,9].

Major muscular effort induces an important energetic consumption: ¾ of this energy is converted into heat. If exercise is practised at the heat, thermoregulation may be more easily overloaded: asymptomatic muscular hyperthermia may develop and reach 41°, inducing tissue damages, in particular of muscle fibres, accentuated by anaerobic metabolism of muscles and lactic acid production. This increase in core temperature has to be counteracted by thermoregulatory processes, as global cutaneous vasodilatation and sweating.

Prolonged effort may induce an exhaustion of calf muscles and a diminution of the efficacy of venous return. Long walking or running induces an important diminution of venous filling time [7]. Decrease of venous drainage results in venous stasis, even in venous healthy individuals, which may induce erythrocytes extravasation, purpura, and vasculitis.

Patients suffering from lipedema are prone to a lesser venous drainage and orthostatic oedema. As these characteristics are hereditary, it does not astonish that one female patient mentioned similar events occurring in her sister. Patients with lipedema are not usually athletic and their muscles are then more rapidly exhausted. The accumulation of fat on the legs may also limit transcutaneous heat elimination and increase core temperature in the muscles at exercise. Those 2 facts may favour EIV and explain the predominance of females in several observations [1-3,11,12].

EIV occurring in hikers in hot climate, mostly females, after an unusual effort, should be distinguished from EIV observed in marathon participants, close to exhaustion, with risks of major complications (severe biological troubles, occult digestive blood loss, up to potentially fatal colic ischemia).

Clinical Aspect

Erythematous, urticarial, or purpuric plaques (figures 1,2,3) arise at the medial lower leg after prolonged and unusual effort in warm climate. The flare is generally sharply delimited at its lower part, not involving skin compressed by socks, but may occasionally extend into the retromalleolar groove, at the dorsum of the foot, or spread to the thigh. Intensity of the eruption depends on heat, and exercise intensity. Lesions are more severe in patients suffering from oedema, with predominance on the oedematous side, if unilateral.

Patients mainly complain of itch, pain, or burning sensation. There is neither systemic repercussion nor abdominal pain, as can be observed in marathonians.

The flare spontaneously resolves in 3 - 10 days, depending on the importance of the eruption.

Relapses are frequent, mostly triggered by similar factors (walking, climbing, and hot weather). Induction of EIV may be very specific. In one of our patients, EIV occurred only when walking in the mountains, never in flat country [3]. In others, the flare happened only when wearing badly adapted shoes. Some patients did not experience relapses, as they spontaneously limited their activities at the hot season to avoid a new flare.

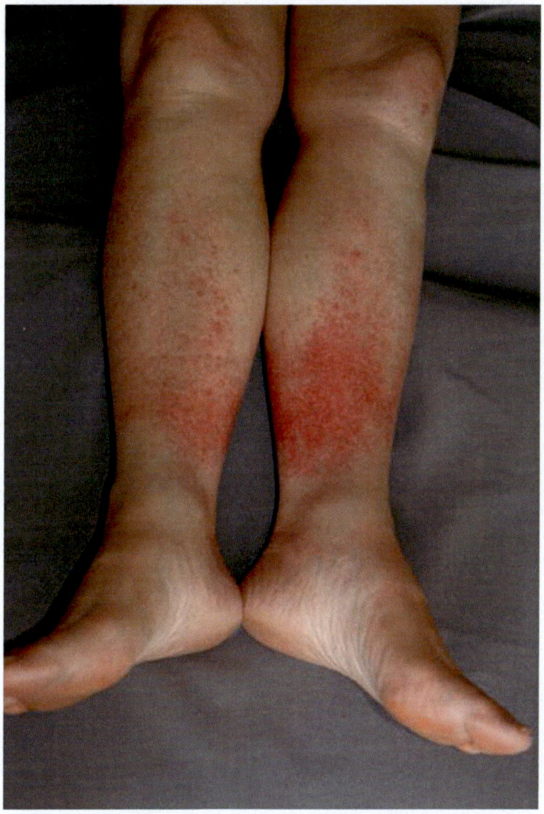

Figure 1. Bilateral asymetric erythematous and purpuric flare of the medial lower leg. The linear inferior bordure corresponds to the pressure exerted by the socks.

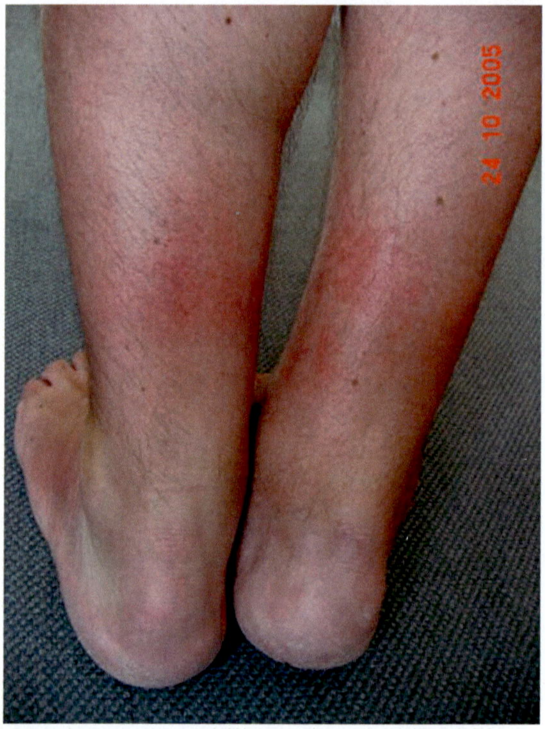

gure 2. Bilateral erythematous flare of the medial and posterior lower leg, with a sharp delimitation of inferior portion.

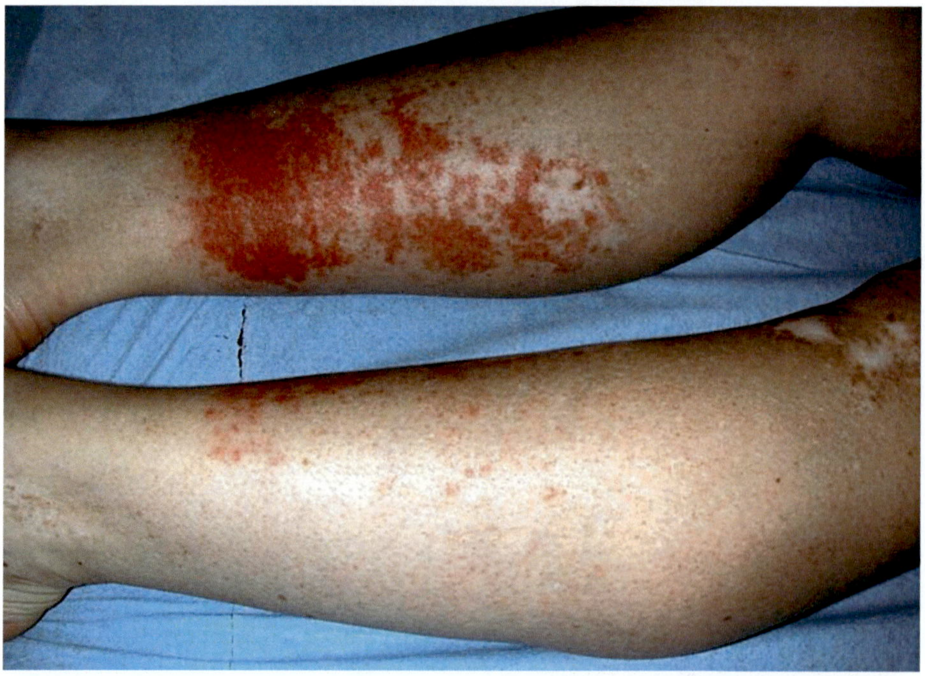

Figure 3. Typical erythematous and purpuric flare of the medial lower leg. The flare spares the scar of the upper medial part of the leg.

Association to other Disorders

We observed lipedema (type Allen Hines) in all of our female patients (presently more than 50), who were also prone to orthostatic oedema.

No clear cut relation with chronic venous disorder (CVD) was established. 80% of our patients who underwent complete vascular investigations with duplex utrasound presented no clinical signs (class C_0 of CEAP classification), or only minor signs (C_1) of CVD. Stripping of one incompetent saphenous vein (C_2) did not prevent relapses of EIV, which recurred regularly since the operation. EIV was bilateral in 1 patient, although saphenous incompetence was unilateral [3].

Investigations

Blood investigations, including blood count, or even electrophoresis, C3, C4 in some patients, were not relevant. Research for antinuclear antibodies was negative. All patients were healthy, without any particular history or routine blood test abnormalities during the last years. Long lasting history of EIV (up to 10 years in several patients) suggests exclusion of any serious underlying pathology.

When performed [2,3,9], histology assessed moderate leucocytoclastic vasculitis (perivascular lymphocytic and neutrophilic infiltrates with some eosinophils, nuclear dust, purpura, œdema and thickening of the vessel walls, with occasional fibrinoid degeneration), or urticarial vasculitis. The microscopic aspect may depend on the delay between the onset of the eruption and the biopsy, which varied between one and 2 days. In marathon participants, direct immunofluorescence revealed deposits of C3 along capillaries endothelial cells, and in few patients granulous deposits of IgM in capillary walls [9].

Treatment

Treatment is not mandatory as EIV fades spontaneously. Topical steroids may help in relieving symptoms.

Compression (if well fitted) may be effective in preventing new flares, as topical application of steroids on the legs one hour before the exercise, prednisone intake, injection of long acting systemic steroids, or oedema protective agents [2,3,11,12].

Occasional effect of manual lymphatic drainage may demonstrate the influence of lipedema on EIV.

Conclusion

The clinical picture of EIV is typical and easy to recognize: relapsing, erythematous, urticarial or purpuric, pruriginous flare of the leg, with a distal linear limit, occurring immediately after an unusual effort in hot climate.

EIV is not uncommon both in hikers and in marathon runners, although not yet mentioned in textbooks. This only recently described entity should be known of specialists concerned by exercise in women.

REFERENCES

[1] Ramelet AA. Vasculite d'effort. *Ann. Dermatol. Venereol.* 2003 ; 130 : 1194

[2] Ramelet AA. Exercise induced purpura. *Editorial. Dermatology.* 2004; 208:293-296

[3] Ramelet AA. Exercise induced vasculitis. *JEADV.* 2006; 20: 423-427

[4] Ramelet AA, Monti M. *Phlebology, the Guide,* page 154. Paris : Elsevier, 1999

[5] Ramelet AA, Kern P, Perrin M. *Varicose veins and telangiectasias,* page 86. Paris, Elsevier, 2004

[6] Ramelet AA, Perrin M, Kern P, Bounameaux, *Phlébologie,* 5th ed., page 160. Paris, Masson, 2006

[7] Veraart JCJM, Prins M, Hulsmans RFHJ, Neumann HAM. Influence of endurance exercise on the venous refilling time of the leg. *Phlebol.* 1994; 23: 120-123

[8] Veraart JCJM, Prins M, Neumann HAM. Effet d'une marche de 80 km sur le système veineux. *Phlébologie.* 1995; 48: 429-431

[9] Prins M, Veraart JCJM, Vermeulen AHM, Hulsmans RFH, Neumann HAM. Leucocytoclastic vasculitis induced by prolonged exercise. *Brit. J. Dermatol.* 1996; 134: 915-918

[10] Kelly RI, Opie J, Nixon R. Golfer's vasculitis. *Australas J. Dermatol.* 2005;4611-4.

[11] Mathelier-Fusade P. Amsler E., Leynadier F.. Dermite des marcheuses : nouvelle entité ? Poster. *Ann. Dermatol. Venereol.* 2003;130:4S160

[12] Pouaha J, Toussaint P, Cholez C, Rigon J, Vilain M, Panterbrick B, Cuny J. Purpura induit par l'effort. Poster. *Ann. Dermatol. Venereol.* 2004 ; 131 :1 S211-212

In: Exercise and Women's Health
Editor: Laura A. Charlington, pp. 17-24
ISBN: 978-1-60456-013-8

Short Communication

IRON NUTRITION AND THE FEMALE ATHLETE

James P. McClung*

Military Nutrition Division; United States Army Research Institute of Environmental Medicine; Natick, MA 01760

ABSTRACT

Iron is a nutritionally essential trace element that functions through incorporation into proteins and enzymes. Many of these proteins and enzymes, including hemoglobin, myoglobin, and cytochrome c, are essential for energy metabolism and physical performance. Iron deficiency affects a significant number of premenopausal women, due mainly to the combination of low dietary intake and iron losses through menstruation. It has been reported that the prevalence of iron deficiency is especially high in female athletes. Iron deficiency is associated with a series of negative consequences, including fatigue, diminished maximal work capacity, impaired aerobic adaptation, and reduced energetic efficiency. This chapter will focus on the effects of diminished iron status on performance in the female athlete. Potential causes of iron deficiency, including diet, impaired iron absorption, and increased whole body turnover will be addressed. Furthermore, the potential benefit of iron supplementation for certain female athletes will be discussed, to include a review of the available literature regarding iron supplementation and physical performance.

INTRODUCTION

Iron is a nutritionally essential trace element that is required for life. The importance of iron for human health was first discovered in the early eighteenth century when it was found that iron was a major constituent of human blood (McCollum, 1957; Yip and Dallman, 1996). Subsequently, in 1832, iron tablets were provided to young women with what was described as deficient "coloring matter" in blood (Yip and Dallman, 1996), and in 1932 it was demonstrated for the first time that iron could be used for the synthesis of hemoglobin (Heath

* James P. McClung: James.McClung@na.amedd.army.mil

et al., 1932). Since then, the biochemical roles of iron in the body have been well described. Iron is a known component of many proteins and enzymes besides hemoglobin, including myoglobin, cytochrome c, NADH dehydrogenase, and succinate dehydrogenase. Many of these proteins and enzymes are essential for the maintenance of energy metabolism and the optimization of human performance.

Despite advanced understanding of the important roles of iron in the body, iron deficiency and iron deficiency anemia remain prevalent in both the developed and developing world. In fact, iron deficiency is the most prevalent micronutrient deficiency disease in the world (DeMaeyer and Adiels-Tegman, 1985; Stoltzfus, 2001). In the United States, recent data suggests that iron deficiency affects up to 16% of females between the ages of 16-19 years, and iron deficiency anemia affects up to 4% of females between the ages of 20-49 years (Looker et al., 2002). Iron deficiency and iron deficiency anemia tend to affect young women more often than men because of the combination of low dietary iron intake and the natural loss of blood that occurs through menstruation. Because of the high prevalence of iron deficiency and iron deficiency anemia in premenopausal women, and the role of iron nutrition in energy metabolism and performance, this chapter will focus of the importance of iron nutrition for the female athlete.

IRON NUTRITION

Iron appears in common foods in two forms: heme and non-heme. Heme iron is typically found in meat sources and is more available for absorption than non-heme iron, which is found in foods of vegetable origin. It is estimated that the rate of absorption of heme iron may range from 15 to 35%, whereas the rate of non-heme absorption may only be from 2 to 20% (Monsen, 1988). The rate of absorption of iron is affected by a number of factors, including the levels of iron stores and the effect of dietary promoters and inhibitors of non-heme iron absorption. Inhibitors of non-heme iron absorption found in common foods include tannins, found in coffee and tea, and phytate, found in wheat germ and bran. Enhancers of non-heme iron absorption include ascorbic acid (vitamin C) and factors in meat, which are known to improve non-heme iron absorption when meat products are consumed during a meal. Sources of heme iron include organ meats, beef, mollusks (such as oysters and clams), and dark meats from poultry sources. Sources of non-heme iron include leafy green vegetables (such as spinach and collard greens), nuts, and beans. Other good sources of iron include fortified or enriched foods, such as breakfast cereals and certain enriched bread products. In fact, some common fortified ready-to-eat cereals contain the entire dietary recommended intake (DRI) for iron in one serving. The iron content of some common food sources appear in table 1.

The most recent DRIs for iron are 15 mg/day for girls between the ages of 14-18 years and 18 mg/day for women between the ages of 19-50 years (IOM, 2001). The DRI for pregnant women is higher, 27 mg/day, due to the gestational needs of the fetus and the blood losses that occur during delivery (IOM, 2001). The DRI for boys ages 14-18 years is 11 mg/day, and the recommendation for men 19 years and over is 8 mg/day (IOM, 2001). The DRI is lower for males because of the lack of iron loss through menstruation. For female athletes, a number of important factors affecting iron nutrition should be considered. First, female athletes that are vegetarian or vegan need to consider compounds found in vegetable products that inhibit iron absorption. With vegetarian or vegan diets the lack of heme iron coupled with high phytate content may contribute to diminished iron absorption. Female athletes who may be actively trying to lose weight or maintain a certain body weight may tend to avoid foods that are high in heme iron, such as red meats, which could also impact iron status.

Table 1. Iron content of common foods

Food	Serving Size	Iron Content (mg)
Beans (pinto, boiled)	1 cup	3.57
Beef (ground, broiled)	3 oz.	2.01
Beef (top sirloin, broiled)	3 oz.	1.47
Bread (white, toasted)	1 slice	0.73
Cereal (ready-to-eat, TOTAL corn flakes)	1-1/3 cup	18.00
Chicken (breast, no skin, roasted)	1/2 breast	0.89
Clams (mixed species, raw)	3 oz.	11.88
Collards (boiled)	1 cup	2.20
Egg (whole, raw)	1 large	0.92
Fish (tuna, canned, drained)	3 oz.	0.82
Milk (1% milkfat, fluid)	1 cup	0.07
Nuts (almonds)	1 oz.	1.22
Pork (loin, broiled)	3 oz.	0.68
Raisins (seedless)	1 cup	2.73
Spinach (drained, boiled)	1 cup	6.43
Tomato (red, raw)	1 tomato	0.33
Wheat flour (whole grain)	1 cup	4.66
Yogurt (plain, low fat)	8-oz. container	0.18

Adapted from the USDA National Nutrient Database for Standard Reference, Release 17.

Iron Balance

A number of factors influence iron balance in humans. Iron balance is determined by the net difference between the amount of iron that is excreted and the amount of iron that is absorbed from the diet. Paramount for maintaining iron balance is the consumption of adequate levels of iron through the diet in bioavailable forms. Although a small amount of iron is excreted regularly in urine and feces, menstruation imparts a significant loss of iron in the female athlete (Hallberg et al., 1966; Milman et al., 1998). In fact, menstrual blood loss is a strong predictor of iron status (Harvey et al., 2005), and female athletes with high menstrual losses may be especially prone to iron deficiency. On the other hand, while it is possible that the development of amenorrhea in certain populations of females may protect against depleted iron stores (Swenne, 2007), the relationship between amenorrhea and iron status is not well understood. Female athletes may also excrete iron through a number of other mechanisms, including blood donation, gastrointestinal bleeding, and sweat loss. Some of the factors contributing to the maintenance of iron balance appear in figure 1.

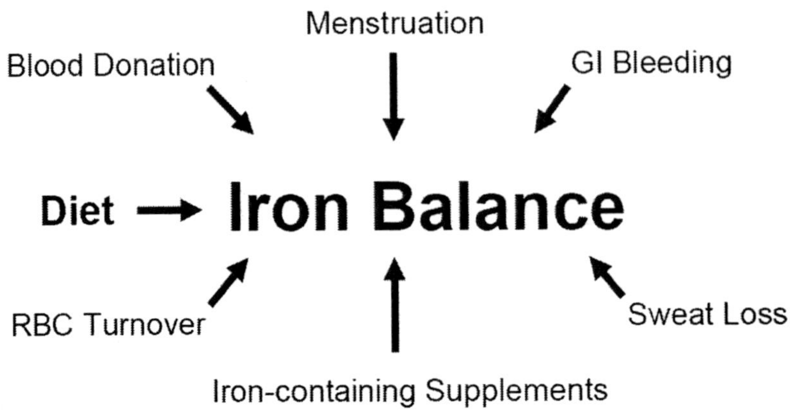

Figure 1. Factors affecting iron balance in the female athlete.

When iron balance is negative, iron deficiency may occur. Iron deficiency occurs in stages, starting with the depletion of iron storage proteins, such as ferritin. When iron storage proteins become depleted, the iron supply to tissues is reduced, as indicated by low serum iron concentrations and diminished saturation of the iron transport protein, transferrin. Iron deficiency anemia may occur if negative iron balance persists. Iron deficiency anemia, the final, and most severe, stage of iron deficiency occurs as prolonged limited serum and tissue iron supply cause diminished production of hemoglobin, which is necessary for oxygen transport. There are a number of functional consequences of iron deficiency anemia. Although the best described consequence of iron deficiency anemia is reduced work performance, other negative consequences include diminished intellectual performance, altered body temperature regulation, reduced immunity and resistance to infections, and adverse pregnancy outcomes (Yip and Dallman, 1996).

Iron Balance in Athletes

The term "sports anemia" first appeared in the literature in 1970 (Yoshimura, 1970). This term refers to diminished hemoglobin concentrations that may occur in response to physical training. This response is often attributed to the plasma volume expansion that occurs during training. Early studies described this effect in male athletes undergoing intensive physical training (de Wijn et al., 1971; Radomski et al., 1980). More recent studies in female athletes participating in endurance exercises have shown that physical training may have a negative effect on not only hemoglobin, but also early indicators of iron status (Reviewed in Beard and Tobin, 2000). For example, in a retrospective review of hematological data collected over 6 years, Ashenden et al. (1998) found that mean serum ferritin levels fell approximately 25% during the training seasons of female rowers, basketball players, and netball players. Another study reported decreased serum iron, total iron binding capacity, and serum ferritin concentrations in female athletes over a 7 week training period (Magazanik et al., 1988). In addition, studies with female Soldiers suggest that physical activity may have a negative effect on iron balance. In American Soldiers, decrements in iron status have been reported upon the completion of the basic combat training (BCT) course (McClung et al., 2006). Activities associated with BCT include aerobic exercises such as tactical road marches, rappelling, and obstacle courses, as well as muscle strength training including callisthenic exercises, push-ups, and sit-ups (Knapik et al., 2002).

Although the exact mechanism by which physical activity (independent of diet and changes in plasma volume) imparts a negative effect on iron balance has not been definitively identified, a number of hypotheses have been proposed. Possible mechanisms include gastrointestinal bleeding after running (Stewart et al., 1984), iron loss through sweat (Brune et al., 1986), increased whole body iron turnover (Ehn et al., 1980), and hematuria as a result of running (Siegel et al., 1979).

The hypothesis that increased gastrointestinal blood loss occurs in runners is supported by the findings of Stewart et al. (1984), who found that fecal hemoglobin levels increased in 20 of 24 runners following a long distance race. Iron losses through urine have also been documented in runners, as hematuria has been observed in up to 18% of athletes immediately following a marathon (Siegel et al., 1979). Increased iron turnover in athletes was observed by Ehn et al. (1980), who found that whole-body loss of isotopic iron occurred approximately 20% more quickly in female athletes as compared to non-athletes.

Iron Balance and Physical Performance

Disruptions in iron balance could have important implications for the female athlete, as reduced physical performance is the best described effect of iron deficiency anemia. The negative effect of iron deficiency anemia on physical performance is due to the important role of iron dependent proteins in maintaining the electron transport chain and oxygen delivery to tissues. For instance, iron deficiency anemia is known to decrease maximal oxygen consumption in proportion to hemoglobin-mediated decreases in oxygen transport capacity (Gardner et al., 1977; Davies et al., 1982). Classical human studies have described reduced physical performance with varying degrees of anemia (Viteri and Torun, 1974; Basta et al., 1979; Edgerton et al., 1979). In one such study, Gardner et al. (1977) measured performance on a multistage treadmill test using a group of female volunteers with varying hemoglobin levels. Data from that study indicated that total time on the treadmill, percentage of volunteers that reached the highest work load (0 versus 100%) and postexercise lactate levels all correlated with hemoglobin levels.

Few studies have investigated the effect of earlier stages of iron depletion on performance in women, although lower maximal oxygen consumption has been reported in iron-depleted women without anemia (Zhu and Haas, 1997). Furthermore, iron repletion is known to increase energetic efficiency in nonanemic women with iron depletion (Zhu and Haas, 1998).

Iron Supplementation

Data from recent iron supplementation trials suggests that there may be some performance benefit to maintaining positive iron balance, even in nonanemic women. In one recent trial, Hinton et al. (2000) provided iron-depleted (low serum ferritin) nonanemic women with daily doses of 100 mg of an iron salt, ferrous sulfate, or placebo, for 6 weeks. The supplement provided approximately 16 mg/day of elemental iron, which is close to the current DRI of 18 mg/day. At the end of the study, the group receiving the iron supplement had improved iron balance, which was measured using a series of iron status indicators, and a decreased time to completion of a 15-km cycle ergometer test. In a subsequent investigation, also studying iron-depleted nonanemic volunteers, individuals who were supplemented daily for 6 weeks with 150 mg of ferrous sulfate (24 mg elemental iron/day) demonstrated increased gross energetic efficiency (ratio of energy expended to work performed) during a submaximal exercise test (Hinton and Sinclair, 2007). Similar placebo controlled double-blind trials have demonstrated improved iron status and increased maximal oxygen uptake and endurance capacity after 6 weeks of iron supplementation at similar levels (16 mg iron/day; Brownlie et al., 2002; 2004).

When considering iron supplements for the female athlete a number of factors should be addressed, including dose, frequency, and potential side effects. The health of the athlete should be the main consideration. First, supplements above the tolerable upper intake level (UL) set forth by the Institute of Medicine are not recommended. The UL for adults (male and female) is 45 mg/day (IOM 2001). Certain populations, including those with iron storage disorders, such as hemochromatosis, should not consume iron supplements. Furthermore, high dose iron supplements have been associated with a number of side effects, including constipation, nausea, and vomiting (Hallberg et al., 1966). In cases where athletes have been diagnosed as iron deficient by a medical professional, a low dose (10-20 mg/day) supplement with a highly bioavailable iron salt, such as ferrous sulfate, should be considered.

Conclusion/Recommendations

Avoiding the negative effects of poor iron balance is critical for optimizing the performance of the female athlete. Female athletes may become iron deficient due to the consumption of foods that are low in iron or contain inhibitors of iron absorption. Physical activity itself may have a negative impact on iron balance. As such, female athletes should focus on consuming DRI levels of iron (18 mg/day for premenopausal women) through meals rich in bioavailable iron sources, such as meats and fish. Vegetarian female athletes should consume iron rich foods such as spinach or beans, as well as iron enriched or fortified foods, such as ready-to-eat cereals. In cases where iron deficiency or iron deficiency anemia have been diagnosed by a physician, the female athlete may consider the use of low dose iron supplements under the supervision of appropriately trained medical or dietary professionals.

Disclaimer

The opinions or assertions contained herein are the private views of the authors and are not to be construed as official or as reflecting the views of the Army or the Department of Defense. Any citations of commercial organizations and trade names in this report do not constitute an official Department of the Army endorsement of approval of the products or services of these organizations.

REFERENCES

Ashenden MJ, Martin DT, Dobson GP, Mackintosh C, and Hahn AG. (1998) Serum ferritin and anemia in trained female athletes. *Int. J. Sport Nut. Ex. Metab,* 8:223-9.

Basta SS, Soekiman MS, Karyadi D, and Scrimshaw NS. (1979) Iron deficiency anemia and the productivity of adult males in Indonesia. *Am. J. Clin. Nutr,* 32:916-25.

Beard J and Tobin B. (2000) Iron status and exercise. *Am. J. Clin. Nutr,* 72:594S-7S.

Brownlie T IV, Utermohlen V, Hinton PS, Giordano C, and Haas JS. (2002) Marginal iron deficiency without anemia impairs aerobic adaptation among previously untrained women. *Am. J. Clin. Nutr,* 75:734-42.

Brownlie T IV, Utermohlen V, Hinton PS, and Haas JD. (2004) Tissue iron deficiency without anemia impairs adaptation in endurance capacity after aerobic training in previously untrained women. *Am. J. Clin. Nutr,* 79:437-43.

Brune M, Magnusson B, Persson H, and Hallberg L. (1986) Iron losses in sweat. *Am. J. Clin. Nutr,* 43:438-43.

Davies KJ, Maguire JJ, Brooks GA, Dallman PR, and Packer L. (1982) Muscle mitochondria bioenergetics, oxygen supply, and work capacity during dietary iron deficiency and repletion. *Am. J. Physiol,* 242:E418-27.

de Wijn JF, de Jongste JC, Mosterd W, and Willebrand D. (1971) Hemoglobin, packed cell volume, serum iron, and iron binding capacity of selected athletes during training. *J. Sports Med,* 11:42-51.

DeMaeyer E and Adiels-Tegman M. (1985) The prevalence of anemia in the world. *World Health Stat. Q,* 38:306-16.

Edgerton VR, Gardner GW, Ohirya Y, Gunawardena KA, and Senewiratne B. (1979) Iron-deficiency anemia and its effect on worker productivity and activity patterns. *Br. Med. J,* 2:1546-9

Ehn L, Carlmark B, and Hoglund S. (1980) Iron status in athletes involved in intense physical activity. *Med. Sci. Sports Exerc,* 12:61-4.

Gardner GW, Edgerton VR, Senewiratne B, Barnard RJ, and Ohira Y. (1977) Physical work capacity and metabolic stress in subjects with iron deficiency anemia. *Am. J. Clin. Nutr,* 30:910-7.

Hallberg L, Hogdahl AM, Nilsson L, and Rybo G. (1966) Menstrual blood loss and iron deficiency. *Acta Med. Scand,* 180:639-50.

Hallberg L, Ryttinger L, and Solvell L. (1966) Side-effects of oral iron therapy. A double-blind study of different iron compounds in tablet form. *Acta Med. Scand. Suppl,* 459:3-10.

Harvey LJ, Armah CN, Dainty JR, Foxall RJ, Lewis DJ, Langford NJ, and Fairweather-Tait SJ. (2005) Impact of menstrual blood loss and diet on iron deficiency among women in the UK. *Br. J. Nutr,* 94:557-64.

Heath CW, Strauss MB, and Castle WB. (1932) Quantitative aspects of iron deficiency in hypochromic anemia. *J. Clin. Invest,* 11:91-110.

Hinton PS, Giordano C, Brownlie T, and Haas JD. (2000) Iron supplementation improves endurance after training in iron-depleted, nonanemic women. *J. Appl. Physiol,* 88:1103-11.

Hinton PS and Sinclair LM. (2007) Iron supplementation maintains ventilatory threshold and improves energetic efficiency in iron-deficient nonanemic athletes. *Eur. J. Clin. Nutr,* 61:30-9.

Institute of Medicine. (2001) Iron, In: *Dietary Reference Intakes.* National Academy Press, Washington DC, pp 290-393.

Looker AC, Cogswell ME, and Gunter MT. (2002) *Iron deficiency* – United States, 1999-2000. MMWR Morb Mortal Wkly Rep, 51:897-9.

Knapik JJ, Canham-Chervak M, Hauret K, Laurin M, Hoedebecke E, Craig S, Montain SJ. (2002) Seasonal variations in injury rates during US Army basic combat training. Ann. Occup. Hyg, 46:15-23.

Magazanik A, Weinstein Y, Dlin RA, Derin M, Schwartzman S, and Allalouf D. (1988) Iron deficiency caused by 7 weeks of intensive physical exercise. *Eur. J. Appl. Physiol,* 57:198-202.

McClung JP, Marchitelli LJ, Friedl KE, and Young AJ. (2006) Prevalence of iron deficiency and iron deficiency anemia among three populations of female military personnel in the US Army. *J. Am. Coll. Nutr,* 25:64-9.

McCollum EV. (1957) *A history of nutrition. Houghton Mifflin,* Boston, pp 334-358.

Milman N, Clausen J, and Byg KE. (1998) Iron status in 268 Danish women aged 18-30 years: influence of menstruation, contraceptive method, and iron supplementation. *Ann. Hematol,* 77:13-9.

Monsen ER. (1988) Iron nutrition and absorption: Dietary factors which impact iron bioavailability. *J. Am. Diet Assoc,* 88:786-90.

Radomski MW, Sabiston BH, and Isoard P. (1980) Development of "sports anemia" in physically fit men after daily sustained submaximal exercise. *Aviat. Space Environ. Med,* 51:41-5.

Siegel AJ, Hennekens CH, Solomon HS, and Van Boeckel BV. (1979) Exercise-related hematuria: findings in a group of marathon runners. *JAMA,* 241:391-2.

Stewart JG, Ahlquist DA, McGill DB, Ilstrup DM, Schwartz S, and Owen RA. (1984) Gastrointestinal blood loss and anemia in runners. *Ann. Intern. Med,* 100:843-5.

Stoltzfus RJ. (2001) Defining iron-deficiency anemia in public health terms: time for reflection. J Nutr, 131:565S-567S.

Swenne I. (2007). Haematological changes and iron status in teenage girls with eating disorders and weight loss-the importance of menstrual status. *Acta Paediatr,* 96:530-3.

Viteri FE and Torun B. (1974). Anemia and physical work capacity. *Clin. Hematol,* 3:609-26.

Yip R and Dallman PR. (1996) Iron, In: *Present Knowledge in Nutrition.* ILSI Press, Washington DC, pp 277-92.

Yoshimura H. (1970) Anemia during physical training (sports anemia). *Nutr. Rev,* 28:251-3.

Zhu YI and Haas JD. (1997) Iron depletion without anemia and physical performance in young women. *Am. J. Clin. Nutr,* 66:334-41.

Zhu YI and Haas JD. (1998) Altered metabolic response of iron-depleted nonamenic women during a 15-km time trial. *J. Appl. Physiol,* 84:1768-75.

In: Exercise and Women's Health
Editor: Laura A. Charlington, pp. 25-44
ISBN: 978-1-60456-013-8

Chapter 1

OLDER WOMEN'S PERCEPTIONS OF PHYSICAL ACTIVITY: 'DO THEY MATTER?'

***Jane Sims*[*,1], *Colette Browning*[1] *and Deborah Mullins*[2]**
[1] Monash University, Victoria, Australia
[2] Private Consultant, Physiotherapy Educator and Victoria, Australia

ABSTRACT

This chapter examines the perceptions of, and attitudes towards physical activity in older women, focusing upon the findings of structured face to face interviews conducted with a small sample of older Australian women. The women also completed an 'attitudes to physical activity questionnaire' and a one week activity diary. The data were analysed using content analysis techniques. The older women held various interpretations of the term 'physical activity' and these interpretations influenced their attitudes towards physical activity and actual reported behaviour. These perceptions need to be borne in mind when promoting physical activity amongst older women, when assessing older womens' readiness to become physically active and in interpreting their responses to questions about physical activity behaviour patterns. The findings are discussed within the context of the international evidence base, highlighting the public health implications for practitioners, policy makers and researchers.

Keywords: Physical activity, ageing, attitudes, exercise, activity, health.

---

* Address for correspondence: Dr Jane Sims; Healthy Ageing Research Unit, School of Primary Health Care; Monash University; Building 1, 270 Ferntree Gully Road; Notting Hill Victoria 3168 Australia; T: +61 3 9501 2436; F: +61 3 8575 2233; Email: jane.sims@med.monash.edu.au

INTRODUCTION

With an ageing population, planners are looking to strategies to ensure that people age well and productively and promoting healthy ageing is now firmly on the policy agendas of most countries (World Health Organisation, 1997; World Health Organization, 2002). Typically, age-related changes that reduce healthy ageing include decreases in mobility, muscle power and strength. These age-related changes are associated with declines in functionality, reduced independence, increased disability and increased risk of injury and joint stiffness (Buckwalter and Lane, 1997). Evidence is now accumulating that inactivity in later life contributes to disability associated with ageing. For example, Melillo and colleagues note that many conditions ascribed to ageing are actually due to disuse (Melillo et al., 1996).

Physical activity promotion is one strategy to address these age-related changes that is particularly pertinent for older people. Even when physical activity is adopted late in life it is beneficial. A large US study showed that those most active were twice less likely to die with a disability than the inactive (Leveille, Guralnik, Ferrucci, and Langlois, 1999). Research has shown that physical activity is beneficial even in frail older people (Fiatarone et al., 1994), with the exception of those with unstable medical conditions. The individual benefits of physical activity are well established: lower incidence of hypertension, heart disease, osteoporosis, degenerative arthritis, colonic cancer and diabetes mellitus, improved mood and memory function, and a better maintained social network (Mazzeo and Tanaka, 2001). Promoting physical activity in older women is particularly important as the rates of disability in older women consistently exceed the rates in older men, particularly in the old-old cohorts (Australian Institute of Health and Welfare, 2006; Von Strauss, Aquero-Torres, Kareholt, Winblad, and Fratiglioni, 2003). In addition, population-based studies have shown that older women have lower levels of physical activity than older men (Booth, Owen, Bauman, Clavisi, and Leslie, 2000).

At present, women make up a greater proportion of the ageing population (Population Reference Bureau, 2000), although this is set to change as their male counterparts live longer (Australian Bureau of Statistics, 2001). As other commentators have noted, women will not only live longer, they will play a greater role in the workforce, in addition to contributing to the informal care of partners with chronic conditions and to the care of grandchildren. It is therefore important that countries invest in this human resource by implementing strategies that can optimize the health of older women. Physical activity promotion is one such strategy and forms the basis for the discussion in this Chapter.

Current figures from several international surveys demonstrate that older people are less active than other adults (Bauman et al., 2003; Bull, Bauman, Bellow, and Brown, 2004; US National Institute of Health Consensus Development Panel on Physical Activity and Cardiovascular Health, 1996). Population and cohort studies demonstrate progressively declining activity levels at both the population and individual levels (Armstrong and Morgan, 1998; Bauman and Owen, 1999; Bennett, 1998) .While older people are generally aware that physical activity produces health benefits, like other age groups, they express barriers to its adoption (Cohen-Mansfield, Marx, and Guralnik, 2003). The challenge lies in translating the older person's knowledge about the benefits of physical activity into behaviour change in their daily lives.

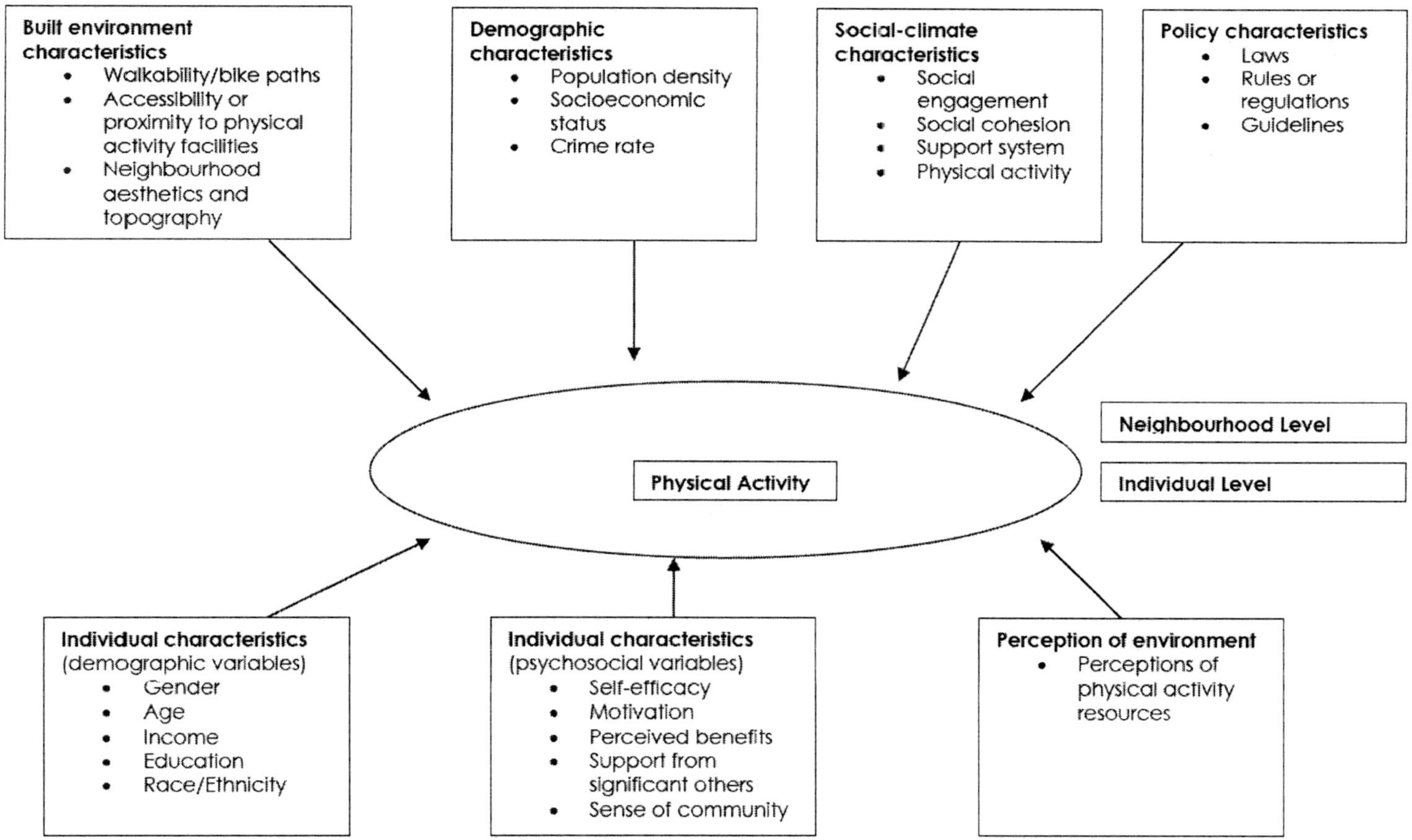

Figure 1. A heuristic multilevel model of influences on physical activity
Source: Adapted from Li, Fisher, Bauman, Ory, Chodzko-Zajko, Harmer, Bosworth and Cleveland, 2005..

Li and colleagues' heuristic multilevel model of influences on physical activity illustrates that factors operating at the individual, societal and structural levels mediate physical activity behaviour in older people (Li, Fisher, and Brownson, 2005). While the role of extrinsic factors such as access to suitable environments for physical activity is important in the adoption and maintenance of physical activity, researchers have recently re-emphasised the key role of intrinsic, personal factors such as attitudes in predicting physical activity patterns (Ball, 2006). These individual level factors are the focus of this Chapter.

There is limited information capturing the older person's perspective about perceived barriers to physical activity: much of the evidence base relates to the general adult population. Intrinsic barriers to physical activity include poor health status, negative attitudes to physical activity, and low motivation and low self efficacy to engage in physical activity (Trost, Owen, Bauman, Sallis, and Brown, 2002). For older people, as with other age groups, a key attitudinal barrier is lack of interest: they can be disinterested due to long term sedentary behaviour and negative attitudes to physical activity (Satariano, Haight, and Tager, 2000). Two further intrinsic barriers for older people are concerns about the risks of physical activity for those with existing health problems and attitudes towards age: in one study, 20% of the older people thought that they were too old to exercise (Cohen-Mansfield et al., 2003). These attitudes are difficult to overcome (Hillsdon, Thorogood, White, and Foster, 2002) as today's generations of older people have been exposed to a curative, paternalistic model of healthcare where illness often necessitated bedrest and inactivity and old age was viewed as a time to 'rest' from the rigours of a physically demanding working life. The impact of motivating factors has also not been fully tested in older people, although in one study, analysis of interviews with older people indicated that self efficacy was the most important predictor of all domains of physical activity: intensity, frequency, session duration and months per year of physical activity engagement (Conn, Burks, Minor, and Mehr, 2003).

Whilst there has been some investigation of the role of personal factors in physical activity participation there has been little exploration of older people's definitions of what actually constitutes physical activity and whether there are any gender differences. One would expect that older men and women would endorse different definitions of physical activity given many older women have not had the benefit of regular participation in structured exercise or sport during their adolescence. Strawbridge and colleagues (Strawbridge, Camancho, Cohen, and Kaplan, 1993) (p.608) suggested that '... older men and women approach physical activity in different ways; men do more structured activities like formal exercise, while physically active women are involved with family, peer, or community activities'.

Older Women's Understandings of Physical Activity and Perceived Barriers to Physical Activity: Findings from an Empirical Study

Women often lack the skills and resources to be physically active in older age. In order to explore more fully older women's understandings of physical activity and perceived barriers to physical activity, it is necessary to examine empirical research. In this Chapter, we report on a recent study conducted using a qualitative methodology involving structured interviews and diary completion. The aim of the study was to explore how older women perceive physical activity and how they define and give meaning to the physical activities they participate in throughout their lives.

Theoretical, purposeful sampling was used to recruit a sample of older women from a community based Welfare Association operated by a local government in metropolitan Melbourne, Australia. Participants were chosen to represent both frequent exercisers (those engaging in physical activity at least once a day) and infrequent exercisers (those who were physically active less than once a day) across a range of living conditions, from living alone independently to living in supported accommodation. The 11 participants were aged between 66 and 90 years. Given that the sample size was small, several sources of information were triangulated to increase the analytic power of the study by increasing reliability and authenticity (Sandelowski, 1995).

Data was collected using a face-to-face, semi-structured interview that took place in the participant's place of residence. The interview lasted about 90 minutes and was audio taped. Topics explored included what the participant did in a typical day, definitions of physical activity and what is 'enough' physical activity, the role of physical activity in the participant's life, and factors that influence engagement in physical activity.

Participants also completed two surveys. One survey identified the demographic characteristics of the participant including marital status, living arrangements, number of children and siblings, educational level, health status and socioeconomic status. The other, Terry et al's (Terry, Biddle, Chatzisarantis, and Bell, 1997) Older Persons' Attitudes Toward Physical Activity and Exercise Questionnaire measured attitudes based on degree of agreement with fourteen statements about physical activity. The questionnaire has four subscales: tension release, health promotion, vigorous exercise and social benefits.

A second interview was also conducted to clarify, confirm, or expand on any issues raised in the first interview. The data from this interview were recorded in a personal log. Data from a one-week Activity Diary (the week preceding the second interview), field notes and an interviewer log were also collected for each of the participants. The Activity Diary included a brief description of the activities engaged in during the day, the effort required for each activity, the time spent on each activity and a description of how the participant felt about the activity (such as enjoyable, exhausting, stimulating).

Grounded theory formed the basis of the analysis. The interview transcripts were explored using an inductive analytical method with emerging themes and concepts coded and analysed. Data triangulation was achieved by comparing interview transcripts with data from the Activity Diary and data from the attitudes questionnaire. Selected quotations are included below to illustrate key themes.

The women were a relatively homogenous sample in terms of their sociodemographic characteristics. The mean age of the sample was 77 years. Eight of the women were widowed, 10 had achieved secondary level schooling or better and all but one rated their health as good.

The main themes that emerged from the analysis of the interview transcripts, the Activity Diary and the attitudes questionnaire were:

- What constitutes physical activity?
- How much physical activity is enough?
- Why engage in physical activity?

What Constitutes Physical Activity?

This group of women exhibited considerable variety in their definitions of what constituted physical activity. The two terms 'physical activity' and 'exercise' were often used interchangeably by the women. Participants distinguished between the purpose of the activity as either formal or functional activity. Exercise (formal activity) was seen as planned and structured in format and designed to promote or improve fitness. Functional types of physical activity included household tasks, walking to the shops and gardening. Those women who perceived that they engaged in low amounts of physical activity often did not include functionally based activities when cataloguing physical activity in their interview. Instead they focused on 'formal' exercise and activities outside those activities required for everyday living. This led to some discrepancy between their verbal accounts of physical activity quantity and quality and what was identified in their Activity Diaries. One 78 year old participant commented in her interview:

> "Apart from walking I don't really do any other physical activities".

Yet when questioned in greater detail during the interview and on examination of her activity diary she also attended weekly yoga classes, did all her own house cleaning and gardening, all requiring effort and exertion. Similarly, a 73 year old participant did not consider walking to the shops as exercise.

> "Well I don't call that exercise. Exercise is something you go to, that you do. I mean that's (walking) is just general daywear".

The same woman attended an organized walking group and defined this type of walking as physical activity, even though the degree of effort was not dissimilar to that expended during her walk to the shops.

In contrast, those participants considering themselves physically active would often use functionally based activities to increase their overall daily output. For instance, they would purposively walk the long way around to the shops, or leave the car at home and walk instead:

> "Instead of taking the car out to go shopping …I'll go around the longer way… to give myself just that little bit of extra exercise". (Informant aged 66 years)

The discrepancy between the verbal accounts of physical activity and the diary accounts is similar to the distinction between occupational activity and leisure time activity that is often used when assessing physical activity amongst working adults. Leisure is free time that people have to allocate to pursuits other than those necessary, contracted or committed. Clearly for older women, functionally-based activities also need to be accounted for.

How Much Physical Activity Is Enough?

Participants were asked what they perceived as 'enough' physical activity. The discussion largely focused upon physical activity intensity rather than frequency or duration, with concerns voiced about undergoing activity of vigorous intensity. Many of the women interviewed held back from participating in physical activities that involved the sort of exertion that would make them "huff" or "puff". When asked about vigorous activity a typical comment was:

> "Well I don't need to do that, do I. Or do I!?"

A number of reasons were elicited for not engaging in vigorous physical activity. Health problems were both inhibitors and motivators for physical activity. For example, one informant aged 66 had to reduce the degree of physical activity because of health problems but was motivated to continue at a lower intensity level:

> "I have arthritis in the knees which means I have to exercise on a regular basis. It's all a matter of learning what you can do and what you can't do."

Another informant aged 77 years noted:

> "Well at my age and stage, there's not much you can do except walking, really, is there? "

Based on the activity diary data none of the study participants engaged in vigorous physical activity. They didn't see the need to do so and generally considered it inadvisable. As a 78 year old stated:

> "I pace myself. I think you have to".

Most of the less active informants were not concerned about trying to improve fitness levels, rather they were trying to maintain the status quo. Amongst the more active participants, women were content to engage in light or moderate intensity activity and would feel this sufficient as they were doing more than their less active peer group members. They appeared not to understand that the amount they did may still be insufficient to achieve physical health benefits. Participants were more interested in maintenance of current activity levels than in improvement of health, mobility and independence.

There was confusion about the distinction between being 'busy' and being physically active. As one 85 year old participant who described herself as very active stated:

> " I've always got something to do. Either someone to phone, being secretary....sickies to send cards to and pass messages on to."

While she may have felt active these largely sedentary activities would not contribute to any fitness impact. Similarly, when Crombie and colleagues (Crombie et al., 2004) interviewed older people about physical activity beliefs and behaviour, many thought they were doing enough to stay healthy, but most were actually sedentary.

Brown et al (Brown, Fuller, Lee, Cockburn, and Adamson, 1999) reported that whilst older focus group participants were unsure what was meant by 'adequate' activity, they understood 'vigorous', 'moderate' and 'light' activity. Consistency of use of these terms was displayed in the definitions these older people provided and the associated exercise types.

Participants in Brown's study also noted that many activities could be conducted at varying intensities. Vaz and Bharathi (2004) found that Indian adult men and women rated particular activities as being of differing intensity. Independent of the person's own reported activity levels, women rated the intensity of jogging, walking uphill, carpentry and manual labour significantly higher than men. There were age-related changes in the perception of intensity of physical activities that persisted even after adjustment for overall physical activity patterns. Thus both age and gender differences in assessment of intensity are important in interpreting self-report assessments of physical activity.

Reasons for Participating in Physical Activity: Perceptions of Influences

The two key reasons given for being physically active were to maintain health and independence respectively. The older women informants placed particular importance on independent living: physical activity adoption had a preventative role.

> "... I do not want to be a nuisance to anyone. ...I'd like to be able to be independent. That's all I ask." (Informant aged 73 years)

Self gratification was also an important motivator:

> "I feel I need the exercise. I must do it. I'm selfish". (Informant aged 73 years)

> " ... absolutely positive feelings from doing it ... in feeling good about myself ... I don't like my body to be sloppy ..." (Informant aged 74 years)

The answers to the Older Person's Attitudes Toward Physical Activity and Exercise Questionnaire support the perceived importance of the health benefits of physical activity as a motivator to exercise. In contrast to other studies in the literature (Gill and Overdorf, 1994 ; Kirkby, Kolt, Habel, and Adams, 1999) social interaction was not a primary motivator for engaging in physical activity amongst these older women. 'Health promotion' and 'tension release' emerged as stronger reasons for exercising than social benefits amongst these informants. As one informant aged 74 years explained:

> "I think that when you do some walking you do the walking. You don't stop and start to talk to people. You just walk. Without stopping."

> "I do it for the exercise, just exercise." (Informant aged 74 years).

However, the results of the attitude questionnaire indicated that positive attitudes didn't translate into positive action: similar scores were found for both frequent and infrequent exercisers.

The womens' current behaviour was potentially influenced by not only their attitudes towards physical activity, but also those of their peers, family and society. Both past experience and current circumstances were contextually relevant. Throughout the lives of many of these women, competition in physical activity was non-existent. Team sports and activities were rare and even tennis which was played by several women was, more often than not, described as 'hit and giggle'. Others noted the lack of encouragement and support from their parents and the general social disapproval of young women engaging in sport as they were growing up.

> "But I don't think I was very competitive". (Informant aged 74 years)

> " I learnt along the way. I didn't grow up with it you see, and the majority of my life I had no opportunity of doing it". (Informant aged 77 years)

This group reported only limited parental, sibling, children or partner influence upon their physical activity behaviour patterns. For most of the womens' parents had had a minor influence on attitudes to and engagement in physical activity:

> "They (her parents) weren't active at all, so they didn't encourage me to be active either." (Informant aged 66 years).

> "My mother didn't encourage. I was an only child and she didn't encourage sporting activities at all". (Informant aged 66 years)

Several of the informants had inactive partners who remained rather bemused by the woman's physical activity. Typical comments were:

> "He doesn't want to do it but that doesn't mean I don't have to. He's perfectly happy to sit in his little corner". (Informant aged 66 years)

> "He says – it's raining you are stupid to go for your exercises today. Well I don't know if he is happy or not, he just has to get used to it". (Informant aged 77 years).

This finding is in contrast to other studies where partner support has predicted participants' physical activity behaviour (Umberson, 1992).

Intrinsic and Extrinsic Influences upon Perceptions of Physical Activity

Individual Level Factors

The research reported here has been able to explore many of the factors regarding women's participation in physical activity. General trends and themes have been identified. It is acknowledged that with only eleven informants full saturation may not have been achieved: however, the findings are reflective of those in the wider literature.

Although rates of physical activity decline with age, physically active older people are not necessarily those who are the healthiest (Sims, Hill, Hunt, Haralambous, Brown, Engel et al., 2006): psychosocial factors also play a part. Many cohort studies have shown the strong inverse association between physical activity behaviour and age, independent of actual health status (Armstrong, Bauman, and Davies, 2000; Semanik, 2002). As the current study data demonstrate, older people primarily decide whether or not to be physically active based upon a range of personally held attitudes and beliefs. These in turn can be influenced by the person's social environment and the perceptions of society at large.

We know that the decision to exercise is based upon assessment of chance of success and the perceived importance of exercising, tempered by costs and the inclination to stay sedentary (Phillips, Schneider, and Mercer, 2004). Overall, the respondents' motivators to be physically active were chiefly health related. As promoted by the current national and international guidelines, incidental, routine activity, where physical activity is integrated into daily life is needed to maintain physical activity behaviour (Bull, Bauman, Bellow, and Brown, 2004). This strategy was more apparent amongst the current study's more physically active women. Purposeful physical activity was included quite deliberately into the daily routines. Older women can be reminded about the benefits of incidental activity. Indeed, King has noted that long term adherance to physical activity is enhanced when the person makes physical activity part of their lifestyle (King, 1991). A re-acknowledgement of incidental activity benefits to promote prolonged independence is needed for both older women *and* men, regardless of age.

Although social benefits were not highly ranked by women responding to the questionnaire in the current study, others have reported social motives for activity to be more important in older women than amongst other population groups (Gill and Overdorf, 1994 ; Kirkby et al., 1999). Kirkby and colleagues obtained feedback from older women already in exercise programs and reported that the oldest old (those 75 years and over) are more likely to find the social aspects most motivating.

Social support contributes to the uptake of physical activity, although its relative impact has yet to be fully determined. Whilst the women in the current study did not emphasise the value of social support, Kahn and colleagues reviewed evidence from interventions using a social support model (Kahn et al., 2002). The common aim of these intervention models was to establish and maintain strong social networks to encourage social relationships to engender behaviour change. Across interventions, a buddy system often operated, with people 'contracted' with one another to achieve physical activity targets through companionship. For example, a two year study focused on older, postmenopausal women (50-65 years old) in walking groups and found good levels of compliance with the three miles three times per week schedule (Kriska et al., 1986). Unfortunately the relative impact of other intervention components, such as self monitoring, phone prompts and incentives, was not reported.

As noted earlier, self efficacy has been shown to be instrumental in the adoption and maintenance of physical activity (Dishman and Ickes, 1981). A participant in the current study highlighted this when stating: "I go for me. This is my time…for feeling good about myself". In promoting good health, self-efficacy may well act as a mediator of wellbeing. McCauley and colleagues recently explored predictors of self esteem in a longitudinal data model and found both self efficacy and physical activity status to be significant predictors (McAuley et al., 2005).

One possible reason for giving up physical activity may be the person's limited exposure to different physical activity types. For instance, responses from older women (65-97 years old) in a US study highlighted that most respondents had only experienced one type of physical activity (Conn et al., 2003). It can be hypothesised that over time, the initial enthusiasm for and benefits from one type of physical activity may wane. Encouraging older people to consider a varied 'diet' of physical activity, meeting a range of biopsychosocial needs, may be helpful.

Societal and Cultural Factors

Although an individual needs to decide to become physically active, a range of external factors can increase their motivation to do so.

Both generational and secular influences can shape physical activity patterns. The current generations of older Westernised adults are influenced by historical perceptions about the appropriateness of physical activity behaviour in older people. These generations were exposed to a physically active lifestyle, where the activity was related to occupational and domestic tasks, rather than to active leisure pursuits or sports engagement. Older people have noted the lack of role models in the media and the confusing messages about exercise (Brown et al., 1999). Whilst expectations are changing and being challenged by media campaigns, the older generation and society at large have not wholly embraced the health promotion message that physical activity is useful at any age. This issue is particularly pertinent with regard to older women: society has tended to view physical activity, at least in the form of 'exercise', as more male-oriented behaviour.

Ory and colleagues have commented on the widespread societal stereotyping of older people, which can negate the uptake of physical activity behaviour amongst older people (Ory, Kinney Hoffman, Hawkins, Sanner, and Mockenhaupt, 2003). Even so, women in the current study noted that there were more cues for older people to be physically active in today's society. They had more options than their parents and there was greater peer acceptance of physical activity adoption in older people.

Secular influences are pertinent when comparing perceptions across countries. Barriers and perceptions can depend upon the population studied. For example, Zunft and colleagues found cross-country differences across the European Union (Zunft, Friebe, Seppelt, et al., 1999) and regional differences are also feasible, given intra-national demographic variation (Parks, Housemann, and Brownson, 2003). Interesting findings emerge from a recent population survey conducted in a developing country, namely Brazil (Reichert, Barros, Domingues, and Hallal, 2007). Eleven per cent of the sample interviewed (358) were aged 65 and above (the maximum age was 92 years). The study allowed comparison of the perceptions of and barriers to physical activity amongst Brazilian adults. According to current criteria, less than a third (27%) of the interviewees were sufficiently active,. A dose response was noted, with physical inactivity being strongly related to the number of cited barriers. Lack of time, dislike of exercising, feeling too tired, lack of company and lack of money were the key predictors of physical inactivity across the sample. The prevalence of these barriers was greater than has been reported in developed countries (Zunft et al., 1999). The researchers catalogued peoples' working time in an attempt to distinguish between 'lack of time' as an objective barrier and as a proxy for 'lack of motivation'. They found that those with longer working hours were more inactive in their leisure time. Amongst older people, the barriers of having no-one to exercise with and lack of time to exercise were cited along with fear of injury and lack of interest. Notably, being too old to exercise was the least commonly cited barrier across the sample. Nevertheless, as amongst the Australian older women in the current study, the group aged over 70 were more likely to report being 'too old' as a barrier, reflecting a lack of knowledge of the benefits of physical activity across the lifespan (Booth, Bauman, Owen, and Gore, 1997; Domingues, Araujo, and Gigante, 2004).

Cultural factors can also be apposite, but it is challenging to disentangle them from other identifying personal characteristics. Henderson and Ainsworth report on qualitative research arising from the US based Cross-Cultural Activity Participation (CAPS) study involving African American and American Indian women aged between 40 and 80 years (Henderson and Ainsworth, 2003). In the US, less than a third of women from minority groups engage in sufficient activity to attain health benefits (US National Institute of Health Consensus Development Panel on Physical Activity and Cardiovascular Health, 1996). Although a sizeable minority of the CAPS sample were aged 60 or over, the authors did not specifically focus on the perceptions of the older women: nevertheless, their overall findings are of note. The women viewed physical activity as important for their health, but similar to the Australian women studied, tended to perceive it in terms of structured exercise (in spite of the broad definition used by the researchers). The women were chiefly sedentary, although they were categorized as 'busy', doing many activities. They discussed the time and situational constraints upon being physically active: the chief barrier appeared to be having no distinct plan to be physically active. The ethic of care (caring more about others' needs than their own) both hindered and enabled physical activity participation. Women wanted to remain healthy to support family, but as carers did not always have time for physical activity pursuits. Interviewees had difficulty articulating racial/cultural influences, other than some cultural traditions such as ceremonies. The barriers and enablers mentioned were similar to those in other population groups (e.g., physical tiredness, family needs, transport, weather, facilities). The researchers and interviewees commented that there was scope for some of the barriers, for example, cost, to be counterbalanced by enablers, such as using walking as a free, accessible means of being physically active.

Options for Providing Physical Activity Programs for Older People

There remains scope to assist adoption and maintenance of physical activity amongst older people (Armstrong and Morgan, 1998). The findings from the current study draw attention to the need for tailored advice giving, offering activity choices and flexibility in meeting goals and targets (King, Rijeski, and Buchner, 1998). Group based physical activity also allows instruction and review of technique by a qualified instructor, overcoming some of the safety concerns mentioned above that act as barriers to physical activity in older people (Cohen-Mansfield et al., 2003). Health professionals are increasingly aware of the need to tailor approaches according to a person's stage of change (Browning, Menzies, and Thomas, 2004). Health professionals have a role to play in giving older people not just the knowledge they need in order to do sufficient exercise to obtain health benefits, but also encouraging the confidence to participate. Being properly informed about the benefits of exercise and how programs can be tailored to one's particular health status can overcome some of the barriers to exercise, such as fear of injury or concerns about unpleasant sensations associated with exercise. Using suitably qualified staff will assist older people in starting and maintaining a physical activity regime. Even where most of the activity occurs in the home and the surrounding community rather than at a facility, people will need some support to maintain their activity levels.

Marketing

Clearly the best strategy for promoting physical activity amongst older women is to encourage the adoption and maintenance of physical activity behaviour across the lifespan. People who are already accustomed to being physically active will find it easier to maintain a behaviour pattern than those trying to develop a lifestyle change in later life. Where older women are the target audience, the marketing messages must be appropriate to their perspectives on life. A study commissioned by the UK Women's Sports Foundation explored the perceptions of older women living in rural communities towards physical activity (Douglas and Carless, 2005). As reported in other studies, the women enjoyed social interaction and preferred to exercise with others. Respondents commented on the limitations of current physical activity options and their marketing. They reported that marketing appeared to be targeted to the younger generation, focused on 'exercise regimes' - such as those traditionally offered by the fitness industry- that were 'unappealing' and was framed in wording that was condescending and unwelcoming thus unlikely to reach an already ambivalent audience. Messages about 'future health gains' needs careful consideration with this group: these older women appeared to be attracted by the more immediate functional and social gains that physical activity offers. We agree with the authors' recommendations that physical activity promoters should attract older women by placing a greater focus on free, incidental activities in the womens' natural domestic and social environment, such as walking, housework and dancing. Strategies to offer opportunities for activities with existing and new exercise partners would be helpful.

Program Delivery

There is no clear evidence for any preferred physical activity program delivery mode. It is likely that a range of options, tailored to the individual, will be needed to assist the maintenance of physical activity behaviour (Brown and Lee, 2004). Hillsdon et al's Cochrane review suggests that more consistent effect size estimates emerge from interventions that include professional guidance and self-direction, along with continued professional support (Hillsdon, Foster, and Thorogood, 2005). Cyarto and colleagues' review suggested that the best outcomes for older people were obtained by interventions featuring greater levels of contact plus multiple reinforcement of the physical activity advice and messages (Cyarto, Moorhead, and Brown, 2004). The US-based Activity Counselling Trial (ACT) reported that whilst women showed improved outcomes with more intensive support, this was not so for men (Simons-Morton et al., 2001) . The US CHAMPS study produced programs that accommodated for older peoples' health, activity preferences and local environment. In addition to minimising injury risk, the programs sought to optimise motivation by reducing barriers to activity (Stewart et al., 2001). The researchers used face-to face behavioural counselling and cognitive techniques to encourage older people to use local exercise venues or to develop their own physical activity programs. Participants attended information meetings, planning sessions and monthly workshops. Participants were strongly encouraged to attend at least the initial two workshops, where a walking clinic was offered. To maintain their involvement they received activity diaries, telephone calls, newsletters and physical function assessments. A range of similar models is currently being field tested in the US as part of the National Blueprint program (National Blueprint Program).

In their review of different approaches to increase physical activity, Kahn et al (2002) acknowledge that community-wide campaigns are effective in increasing physical activity behaviour. To influence the social milieu, there has been a wealth of health education campaigns promoting physical activity in many countries. There have been limited analyses of the specific impact of such campaigns on older people's behaviour, although evaluation of a state media campaign during 1999 (the International Year of Ageing) aimed at older Australians (Bauman et al., 2003) indicated a promising influence. In a longitudinal study of two US communities, the 'intervention' community was targeted using paid advertisements, public relations, and community participatory planning. These strategies significantly raised awareness and achieved sustained changes in reported physical activity behaviour amongst sedentary older people (50-65 year olds) (Reger-Nash et al., 2005).

ENVIRONMENTAL LEVEL FACTORS

There is acknowledgement that one's social and physical surroundings can both influence behaviour patterns (Trost, Owen, Bauman, Sallis, and Brown, 2002). The social capital literature provides some evidence of an association between social capital and health status, although the influences upon the older adult population require greater assessment (Li et al., 2005). Communities where social cohesion and connectedness are greater are more likely to provide an environment that promotes physical activity. Such neighbourhoods are more likely to be viewed as safe to walk in. There is more likely to be support to engage in physical activity, be it from an active neighbour or significant other. There will be places to go for physical activity, both indoors and outdoors.

The importance of environmental factors has been reviewed by other authors (Giles-Corti et al., 2005). The potential influence of the built environment upon the walkability of a person's neighbourhood is receiving greater consideration. Factors such as footpaths, aesthetics, local destinations and facilities are thought to influence people's physical activity behaviour (Berke, Koepsell, Moudon, Hoskins, and Larson, 2007). Environmental issues related to older women's physical activity behaviour are briefly considered here. Researchers in the US used data from a longitudinal study of older people, Adult Changes in Thought (ACT) and geographic information system data to assess the extent to which neighbourhood 'walkability' scores predicted physical activity behaviour in older men and women (Berke et al., 2007). Higher walkability scores were associated with significantly greater likelihood of walking for exercise.

The issue of environment is particularly pertinent for older women. Concerns about personal safety and lack of public transport were cited as barriers to physical activity in Douglas and Carless' work (Douglas and Carless, 2005). Humpel and colleagues note gender differences not only in car usage, but also in perceptions of the environment and convenience to destinations (Humpel, Marshall, Leslie, and Bauman, 2004). The 2001 US National Household Travel Survey indicated that older women make fewer daily trips than older men, including walking trips (Collia, Sharp, and Giesbrecht, 2003). Interestingly, King and colleagues showed a positive relationship between the proximity of post offices and golf courses and the physical activity patterns of older women (King et al., 2005). Patterson and colleagues reported that amongst older women, traditional urban neighbourhood environments appeared more conducive to walking to services than newer suburban settings (Patterson and Chapman, 2004).

IMPLICATIONS FOR FUTURE RESEARCH, PLANNING AND POLICY MAKING

Older women's own definitions of what constitutes physical activity can influence the reporting of the amount and intensity of physical activity performed. The findings from our qualitative study and the broader literature demonstrate that we need to use age-specific tools when measuring older peoples' physical activity behaviour as their perceptions of what constitutes physical activity is different from younger groups. The range of methodological limitations to benchmarking activity levels in older people is acknowledged. Many studies have used age neutral population surveys, with questionable face validity for the older age group. There are relatively few tools that have been specifically developed for use with older people and these require further psychometric testing with large, representative samples (Washburn, 2000). The failure to categorise all forms of physical activity when reporting physical activity behaviour has only been partially addressed by the introduction of measurement tools specifically tailored for use with older people (Washburn, 2000). The promotion of physical activity amongst older people needs to re-emphasise the benefits of informal, incidental functional activities (Sims, Hill, Hunt, Haramboulos, Brown, Engel et al., 2006). In the assessment of prevailing physical activity behaviour amongst older people, healthcare providers and researchers alike need to be aware of the individual's perceptions of physical activity and tailor their querying and advice-giving accordingly. Both functional and formal physical activity can contribute to ongoing participation in a physically active lifestyle. Older women and men require clear definitions and guidelines for physical activity and exercise to objectively measure their own contribution on a regular ongoing basis to ensure quantity and quality are sufficient for health benefits.

CONCLUSION

In conclusion, older women's perceptions of physical activity do matter. In this Chapter, we have illustrated how perceptions are shaped by both intrinsic and extrinsic factors. Policy makers and health providers need to continue to accommodate for personal perspectives in the promotion of physical activity.

ACKNOWLEDGEMENTS

The authors would like to thank the participants of the study who graciously shared their time and thoughts providing a detailed insight into the variety and richness of their lives. In addition thanks go to the Welfare Association for providing an entry point to source these participants. This paper is based on data collected as part of a Master of Gerontology degree completed by Deborah Mullins.

REFERENCES

Armstrong, G., and Morgan, K. (1998). Stability and change in levels of physical activity in later life. *Age and Ageing, 27*((S3)), 17-23.

Armstrong, T., Bauman, A., and Davies, J. (2000). *Physical activity patterns of Australian adults: results of the 1999 national physical activity survey*. Canberra: Australian Institute of Health and Welfare.

Australian Bureau of Statistics. (2001). *Australian Social Trends 2001* (No. Catalogue No. 4102, p2 (projection series II)). Canberra: Australian Bureau of Statistics.

Australian Institute of Health and Welfare. (2006). *Life expectancy and disability in Australia 1988-2003*. Canberra: AIHW.

Ball, K. (2006). People, places ... and other people? Integrating understanding of intrapersonal, social and environmental determinants of physical activity. *J. Sci. Med. Sport, 9*(5), 367-370.

Bauman, A., Armstrong, T., Davies, J., Owen, N., Brown, W., Bellew, B., et al. (2003). Trends in physical activity participation and the impact of integrated campaigns among Australian adults, 1997-99. *Australian and New Zealand Journal of Public Health, 27*(1), 76-79.

Bauman, A., and Owen, N. (1999). Physical activity of adult Australians: epidemiological evidence and potential strategies for health gain. *J. Sci. Med. Sport, 2*, 30-41.

Bennett, K. M. (1998). Gender and longitudinal changes in physical activities in later life. *Age and Ageing, 27*((S3)), 24-28.

Berke, E. N., Koepsell, T. D., Moudon, A. V., Hoskins, R. E., and Larson, E. B. (2007). Association of the built environment with physical activity and obesity in older persons. *American Journal of Public Health, 97*(3), 486-492.

Booth, M., Bauman, A., Owen, N., and Gore, C. J. (1997). Physical activity preferences, preferred sources of assistance , and perceived barriers to increased activity aming physically inactive Australians. *Preventive Medicine, 26*, 131-137.

Booth, M., Owen, N., Bauman, A., Clavisi, O., and Leslie, M. (2000). Social-cognitive and perceived environmental influences associated with physical activity in older Australians. *Preventive Medicine, 31*, 15-22.

Brown, W., and Lee, C. (2004). Grandmothers on the move: benefits, barriers and best practice interventions for physical activity in older women. In M. E. Morris and A. M. M. Schoo (Eds.), *Optimizing exercise and physical activity in older people*. Edinburgh: Butterworth Heinemann.

Brown, W. J., Fuller, B., Lee, C., Cockburn, J., and Adamson, L. (1999). Never too late: older people's perceptions of physical activity. *Health Promotion Journal of Australia, 9*, 55-63.

Browning, C., Menzies, D., and Thomas, S. (2004). Assisting health professionals to promote physical activity and exercise in older people. In M. E. Morris and A. M. M. Schoo

(Eds.), *Optimising exercise and physical activity in older people* (pp. 38-62). Edinburgh: Butterworth Heinemann.

Buckwalter, J. A., and Lane, N. E. (1997). Athletics and osteoarthritis. *Am. J. Sports Med, 25*(6), 873-881.

Bull, F. C., Bauman, A., Bellow, B., and Brown, W. (2004). *Getting Australia Active II: an update of evidence on physical activity for health.* Melbourne: National Public Health Partnership.

Cohen-Mansfield, J., Marx, M., and Guralnik, J. M. (2003). Motivators and barriers to exercise in an older community-dwelling population. *Journal of Ageing and Physical Activity, 11*, 242-253.

Collia, D. V., Sharp, J., and Giesbrecht, L. (2003). The 2001 National Household Travel Survey: a look into the travel patterns of older Americans. *J. Safety Research, 34*, 461-470.

Conn, V., Burks, K., Minor, M., and Mehr, D. (2003). Randomized trial of 2 interventions to increase older women's exercise. *American Journal of Health Behavior, 27*(4), 380-388.

Crombie, I. K., Irvine, L., Williams, B., McGinnis, A. R., Slane, P. W., Alder, E. M., et al. (2004). Why older people do not participate in leisure time physical activity: a survey of activity levels, beliefs and deterrents. *Age and Ageing, 33*, 287-292.

Cyarto, E. V., Moorhead, G. E., and Brown, W. J. (2004). Updating the evidence relating to physical activity intervention studies in older people. *Journal of Science and Medicine in Sport, 7*(1 Suppl), 30-38.

Dishman, R. K., and Ickes, W. (1981). Self-motivation and adherence to therapeutic exercise. *Journal of Behavioral Medicine, 4*(4), 421-438.

Domingues, M. R., Araujo, C. L., and Gigante, D. P. (2004). Knowlegde and perceptions of physical exercise in anault urnan poulation in Southern Brazil. *Cad. Saude Publica, 20*, 204-215.

Douglas, K., and Carless, D. (2005). Physical activity perceptions of older women in Cornwall: summary of findings.

Fiatarone, M. A., O Neill, E. F., Ryan, N. D., Clements, K. M., Solares, G., Nelson, M., et al. (1994). Exercise training and nutritional supplementation for physical frailty in very elderly people. *The New England Journal of Medicine, 330*(25), 1769.

Giles-Corti, B., Broomhall, M., Knuiman, M., Collins, C., Douglas, K., Ng, K., et al. (2005). Increasing walking - How important is distance to, attractiveness, and size of public open space? *American Journal of Preventive Medicine, 28*, 169-176.

Gill, K., and Overdorf, V. (1994). Incentives for exercise in younger and older women *J Sports Behaviour, 17*, 87-97.

Henderson, K. A., and Ainsworth, B. E. (2003). A synthesis of perceptions about physical activity among older African American and American Indian women. *Am. J. Public Health, 93*, 313-317.

Hillsdon, M., Foster, C., and Thorogood, M. (2005). Interventions for promoting physical activity. *Cochrane Database of Systematic Reviews*(1).

Hillsdon, M., Thorogood, M., White, I., and Foster, C. (2002). Advising people to take more exercise is ineffective: a randomized controlled trial of physical activity promotion in primary care. *International Journal of Epidemiology, 31*(4), 808-815.

Humpel, N., Marshall, A. L., Leslie, E., and Bauman, A. (2004). Changes in neighbourhood walking are related to changes in perceptions of environmental attributes. *Annals Behavioral Medicine, 27*, 60-67.

Kahn, E. B., Ramsey, L. T., Brownson, R., Heath, G., E., H., Powell, K. E., et al. (2002). The effectiveness of interventions to increase physical activity: A systematic review. *American Journal of Preventive Medicine, 22*, 73-107.

King, A. (1991). Community intervention for promotion of physical activity and fitness. *Exercise and Sports Science Review, 19*, 211-260.

King, A. C., Rijeski, W. J., and Buchner, D. M. (1998). Physical activity interventions targeting older adults: a critical review and recommendations. *American Journal of Preventive Medicine, 15*, 316-333.

King, W., Belle, S. H., Brach, J. S., Simkin-Silverman, L. R., Soska, T., and Kriska, A. M. (2005). Objective measures of neighborhood environment and physical activity in older women. *Am. J. Prev. Med, 28*, 461-469.

Kirkby, R. J., Kolt, G. S., Habel, K., and Adams, J. (1999). Exercise in older women: motives for participation. *Australian Psychologist, 34*(2), 122-127.

Kriska, A., Bayles, C., Cauley, J., LaPorte, R., Sandler, R., and Pambianco, G. (1986). A randomized exercise trial in older women: increased activity over two years and the factors associated with compliance. *Medicine and Science in Sports and Exercise, 18*(5), 557-562.

Leveille, S. G., Guralnik, J. M., Ferrucci, L., and Langlois, J. A. (1999). Ageing successfully until death in old age: opportunities for increasing active life expectancy. *Am. J. Epidemiol, 149*, 654-664.

Li, F., Fisher, J., and Brownson, R. C. (2005). A multilevel analysis of change in neighborhood walking activity in older adults. *Journal of Aging and Physical Activity, 13*(2), 145-159.

Li, F.L., Fisher, J., Bauman, A., Ory, M.G., Chodzko-Zajko, C.W., Harmer, P., Bosworth, M. and Cleveland, M. (2005). Neighbourhood influences on physical activity in middle-aged and older adults: a multilevel perspective. *Journal of Aging and Physical Activity, (13)*, 87-114.

Mazzeo, R. S., and Tanaka, H. (2001). Exercise prescription for the elderly. *Sports Medicine, 31*(11), 809-818.

McAuley, E., Elavsky, S., Motl, R. W., Konopack, J. F., Hu, L., and Marquez, D. X. (2005). Physical activity, self-efficacy, and self-esteem: longitudinal relationships in older adults. *Journals of Gerontology. Series B, Psychological Sciences and Social Sciences 60*(5), P268.

Melillo, K. D., Futrell, M., Williamson, E., Chamberlain, C., Bourque, A. M., MacDonnell, M., et al. (1996). Perceptions of physical fitness and exercise activity amongst older adults. *J Advanced Nursing, 23*, 542-547.

National Blueprint Program. viewed at http://www.activeforlife.info/about_the_program/national_blueprint.html May 2007.

Ory, M., Kinney Hoffman, M., Hawkins, M., Sanner, B., and Mockenhaupt, R. (2003). Challenging aging stereotypes: strategies for creating a more active society. *American Journal of Preventive Medicine, 25*(3 Suppl 2), 164-171.

Parks., S. E., Housemann, R. A., and Brownson, R. C. (2003). Differential correlates of physical activity in urban and rural adults of various socioeconomic backgrounds in the United States. *J. Epidemiol. Community Health, 57*, 29-35.

Patterson, P. K., and Chapman, N. J. (2004). Urban forms and older residents' service use, walking, driving, quality of life and neighborhood satisfaction. *Am. J. Health Promot, 19*, 45-52.

Phillips, E. M., Schneider, J. C., and Mercer, G. R. (2004). Motivating elders to initiate exercise. *Arch. Phys. Med. Rehabil, 85*(7, Suppl 3), S52-S57.

Population Reference Bureau. (2000). *World population datasheet.* Washington DC: Population Reference Bureau.

Reger-Nash, B., Bauman, A., Booth-Butterfield, S., Cooper, L., Smith, H., Chey, T., et al. (2005). Wheeling walks: evaluation of a media-based community intervention. *Family and Community Health, 28*(1), 64-78.

Reichert, F. F., Barros, A. J. D., Domingues, M. R., and Hallal, P. C. (2007). The role of perceived personal barriers to engagement in leisure-time physical activity. *Am. J. Public Health, 97*, 515-519.

Sandelowski, M. (1995). Triangles and Crystals: On the Geometry of Qualitative Research. *Research in Nursing and Health, 18*, 569-574.

Satariano, W. A., Haight, T. J., and Tager, I. B. (2000). Reasons given by older people for limitation or avoidance of leisure time physical activity. *J. Am. Geriatr Soc, 48*(5), 505-512.

Semanik, P. A. (2002). *Determinants of physical activity in older women with rheumatoid arthritis.* Unpublished PhD Thesis, University of Illinois at Chicago, Health Sciences Center, Illinois.

Simons-Morton, D., Blair, S., King, A., Morgan, T., Applegate, W., O'Toole, M., et al. (2001). Effects of physical activity counselling in primary care: The Activity Counselling Trial: A randomised controlled trial. *Journal of the American Medical Association, 286*, 677-867.

Sims, J., Hill, K., Hunt, S., Haralambous, B., Brown, A., Engel, L., Huang, N., Kerse, N., and Ory, M. (2006). National physical activity recommendations for older Australians: Discussion document. Report to the Australian Government Department of Health and Ageing. Melbourne, National Ageing Research Institute.

Stewart, A., Verboncoeur, C., McLellan, B., Gillis, D., Rush, S., Mills, K., et al. (2001). Physical activity outcomes of CHAMPS II: a physical activity promotion program for older adults. *Journals of Gerontology. Series A, Biological Sciences and Medical Sciences 56*(8), M465.

Strawbridge, W. J., Camancho, T. C., Cohen, R. D., and Kaplan, G. A. (1993). Gender differences in factors associated with physical functioning in old age: a 6-year longitudinal study. *Gerontologist, 33*(5), 603-609.

Terry, P. C., Biddle, S. J. H., Chatzisarantis, N., and Bell, R. D. (1997). Development of a test to assess the attitudes of older adults toward physical activity and exercise. *Journal of Ageing and Physical Activity, 2*, 111-125.

Trost, S. G., Owen, N., Bauman, A. E., Sallis, J. F., and Brown, W. (2002). Correlates of adults' participation in physical activity: review and update. *Med. Sci. Sports Exerc, 34*, 1996-2001.

Umberson, D. (1992). Gender, marital status and the social control of health behaviour. *Soc Sci. Med, 34*(8), 907-917.

US National Institute of Health Consensus Development Panel on Physical Activity and Cardiovascular Health. (1996). Physical activity and cardiovascular health. *Journal of the American Medical Association, 276*(3), 241-246.

Vaz, M., and Bharathi, A. V. (2004). Perceptions of the intensity of specific physical activities in Bangalore, South India: implications for exercise prescription. *J. Assoc. Physicians India, 52*, 541-544.

Von Strauss, E., Aquero-Torres, H., Kareholt, I., Winblad, B., and Fratiglioni, L. (2003). Women are more disabled in basic activities of daily living than men only in the very advanced ages: a study on disability, morbidity, and mortality from the Kungsholmen Project. *Journal of Clinical Epidemiology, 56*, 669-677.

Washburn, R. (2000). Assessment of physical activity in older adults. *Research Quarterly for Exercise and Sports, 71*, S79-S88.

World Health Organisation. (1997). Heidelberg guidelines for promoting physical activities among older person. *Journal of Ageing and Physical Activity, 5*, 2-8.

World Health Organization. (2002). *Active aging: A policy framework*. Geneva: World Health Organization.

Zunft, H. J., Friebe, D., Seppelt, B., Widhalm, K., Remaut de Winter, A.M., Vaz de Almeida, M.D., Kearney, J.M., and Gibney, M. (1999). Perceived benefits and barriers to physical activity in a nationally representative sample in the European Union. *Public Health Nutrition, 2*(1A), 153-160.

In: Exercise and Women's Health
Editor: Laura A. Charlington, pp. 45-66
ISBN: 978-1-60456-013-8

Chapter 2

BENEFITS OF PHYSICAL ACTIVITY IN OLDER WOMEN

Alessia Brescianini, Marco Astengo, Alessandro Sona, Eleonora Quagliotti, Elona Horjeti and Mario Bo*
Section of Geriatrics-Departament of Medical and
Surgical Disciplines-University of Turin, Italy
Molinette Hospital-C.so Bramante 88-10126 Turin, Italy

ABSTRACT

The elderly represent a steadily growing proportion of the populations of the industrialized countries. This is particularly true for elderly women and the elderly over 80.

The physiological decline in the function of systems and apparatuses, the high prevalence of polipathology and the consequent increase in frailty and disability seen in the elderly imply increasing health-care and social burdens. The improvement in treatment of many pathologies affecting adults and older adults has brought about consistent increase in life expectancy and survival rates in these age groups. Nonetheless, maintenance of functional performance should be addressed more intensively, especially through life-style interventions and in particular through the implementation of physical activity programmes. Elderly women have a longer life expectancy and are at the same time more susceptible to frailty and functional decline. Thus they should be the main target of such an intervention. Unfortunately strong evidence in this subgroup is still lacking.

The objective of this review is to summarize the evidence about the effects of physical activity and physical exercise on total mortality, cardiovascular risk, obesity, diabetes, chronic diseases, cognitive and functional impairment, disability and quality of life in old women. In order to do so we analyzed meta-analyses, randomized-controlled trials (RCTs), longitudinal studies and non systematic reviews. A total of 18 studies matched our search criteria (2 meta-analyses, 4 RCTs, 8 longitudinal trials and 4 reviews).

* Correspndence to: MarioBo, tel +390116335006,fax +390116961045, e-mail:mario.bo@unito.it

Most of the analyzed studies showed that physical activity and exercise can improve the above-mentioned outcomes in samples of elderly women. The most acknowleged and consistent benefits of physical activity in older women are a longer life expectancy, a decrease, or at least a stabilization, in body weight, a lower incidence of diabetes complications and a lower incidence of functional impairment among the subjects affected by chronic diseases. Also quality of life is improved by physical activity according to most of the considered studies. In conclusion, physical activity can improve health condition and promote functional integrity in elderly women and thus physical activity appears to play a crucial role in the prevention and treatment of geriatric diseases. According to the evidence here revised, physical activity programmes should be implemented not only in the adults but even in the subgroup of elderly women, through educational campaigns or more individualized interventions.

The elderly represent a steadily growing proportion of the populations of the industrialized countries. This is particularly true for the elderly over 80 and women, who have a longer life expectancy. The almost physiological decline in the function of systems and apparatuses that often characterizes ageing, together with the high prevalence and incidence of polipathology, imply increasing health-care and social burdens. Despite the steady improvement in the prevention and treatment of many pathologies affecting the elderly much has still to be done in order to allow larger proportions of the geriatric population to achieve a successful ageing. Thus, health care systems should focus not only on the prevention and treatment of diseases, but should more widely address improvement and maintenance of functional performance. This can be obtained with programs tailored on single subject, when feasible. Lifestyle interventions, especially the implementation of physical activity programs, appear to be particularly suitable means to obtain such goals.

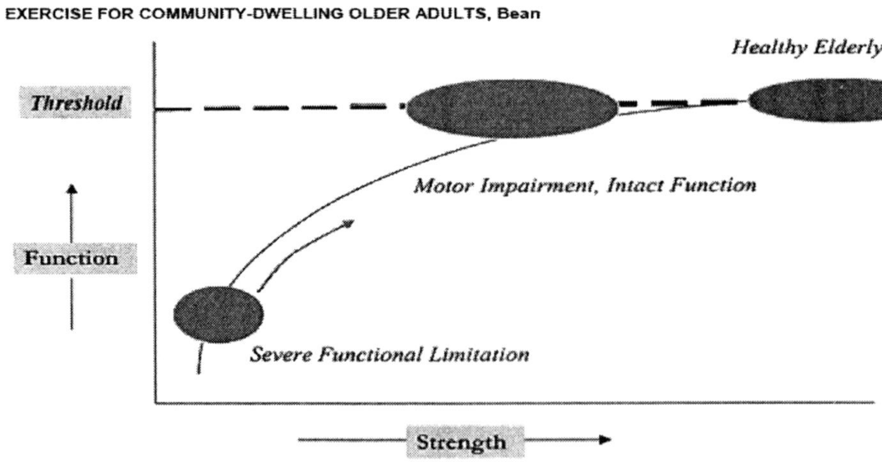

Benefits of exercise for community dwelling older adults;Arch Phys Med Rehabil Vol 85, Suppl 3, July 2004.Jonathan F. bean, MD, MS,Ariona Vora, MD, Walter R.Frontera, MD.

Figure 1. The curvilinear relationship between impairments (ie, reduced strength) and function shows that, at low levels, small increases in strength lead to large increases in function. In contrast, for people at or above the functional threshold (Healthy Elderly), strength improvements have diminishing effects on function; nevertheless; these improvements add to strength reserves, thus augmenting one's resistance to functional decline.

The path from severe functional limitation to functional integrity (Figure 1) can imply substantial social and economical benefits, with increased disability-free life expectation and decreased social burdens.

Old women are more numerous, have a longer life expectancy, and are therefore more prone to develop functional decline and dependency, when compared to men; moreover they are physiologically frailer, have a less favourable body composition, with lower lean mass, and more often fail to see physical activity as a means to obtain wellbeing. For all these reasons, elderly women appear to be the ideal primary target of educational interventions that aim to implement physical activity. Unfortunately strong evidence in this subgroup is still lacking.

Ageing is strongly associated with functional decline and impairment. At the same time the elderly represent an extremely heterogeneous population; this means that for any given age actual "biological age" can vary consistently. The functional status in the elderly mirrors the complex and lifelong interaction between genes and lifestyle. Therefore lifestyle in adulthood becomes a strong predictor of the severity of the functional impairment in late life, yet on the background of a great inter-individual variability. Such a variability can be seen in a number of physiological modifications, which should, thus, be considered age-related rather than age-dependent. This is the case, for example, for the decrease in aerobic capacity and the changes in body composition, with a decline in lean mass, muscular hypotrophy and bone mass reduction.

According to a recent review 32% of the subjects over 70 have some degree of functional limitation while as many as 20% are dependent in at least one activity of daily living (ADL) (Benefits of exercise for Community-Dwelling Older Adyults, Arch Phys Med Rehabil vol 85, suppl3, july 2004, Jonathan F Bean, Ariana Vora, Walter R Frontera). A number of studies have shown how physical activity and fitness directly correlate to survival and quality of life, while an inverse correlation exists with cardiovascular and total morbidity and disability. Constant moderate physical activity appears as important as other preventive measures, weight loss, treatment of hypertension and smoking cessation. This seems to be true in the elderly as well. Physical activity improves aerobic capacity and cardiac performance, lowers blood pressure, and has favourable effects on bone mass and muscular trophism. Progressive Resistance Training (PRT), by means of enhancing both muscular strength and resistance, is thought to be the optimal strategy to achieve function maintenance in both the community-dwelling and institutionalized elderly (Effect of strength and power training on physical function in community-dwelling older adults. J Gerontol A Biol Sci Med Sci 2003;58:171-5. Miszko TA, Cress ME; Slade JM, Covei CJ, Agraval SK Doerr CE).

The aim of this review is to summarize the evidence about the effects of physical activity on total mortality, cardiovascular risk, obesity, diabetes, chronic diseases, cognitive and functional impairment, disability and quality of life in old women. In order to do so we analyzed the available evidence and its strength: meta-analyses and systematic reviews are considered as having the strongest level of evidence, randomized controlled trials (RCT) convey strong evidence, while observational studies represent a good level of evidence.

(questa parte tanto varrebbe copiare dall'articolo!) Physical activity is defined as any movement of the body, that is produced by the contraction of skeletal muscle and that increases energy expenditure compared to the basal; exercise is defined as movements of the body that are organized and repetitive with or without the specific aim of improving physical skills, exercise is considered as a sub-category of physical activity (Exercise comes of age:

rationale and reccomandation for a geriatric exercise prescription. J Gerontol Med Sci 2002; 57:262-82. Fiatarone Singh MA).

Type, intensity and duration of physical activity programmes can vary considerably according to the target population. In order to develop a program of physical activity, that can be effective in improving public health, it is therefore necessary to analyze carefully and critically the type, intensity and duration of physical activity and their relation to clinical outcomes.

In the following Table 1 we summarize some of the definitions of physical activity as reported in some of the analyzed studies.

Table 1.

Study	Definition of physical activity
Miller et al 2000	Physical active: walking 1 mile at least once a week at baseline
Wu et al 1999	Exercise (folk dancing, hiking, jogging, or walking at least twice a week)
Leveille et al 1999	Physical activity: frequency of walking, gardening, and doing vigorous exercise(several times per week; once a week or several times per month; once a month or less)
Huang et al 1998	Physical fitness (total time on a treadmill). Low fitness: lowest 20%; moderate fitness: next 40%; high fitness: next 40% Physical activity. Sedentary: no leisure time physical activity; moderate: some regular leisure-time activity or walking, running, or jogging < 0 miles per week; active: walking, running, or jogging >10 miles per week

Does Late-Life Physical Activity or Exercise Prevent or Minimize Disablement? Am J Prev Med 2003;25:129-136. Julie J. Keysor PhD, PT.

Before engaging in any physical activity program the elderly, especially the ones previously inactive, should undergo a thorough and careful medical visit. Some clinical conditions, in fact, represent an absolute contraindication to physical activity: such are, for example, unstable angina or severe coronary heart disease, end stage heart failure, unstable cardiac dysrhythmias, uncontrolled or poorly controlled hypertension (systolic blood pressure > 200 mmHg, diastolic blood pressure > 110 mmHg), aortic or cerebral aneurysms, recent cerebral bleeding, end-stage systemic diseases, recent eye surgery or retinal hemorrhage, recent soft tissue trauma and advanced dementia (Exercise Standard. A statement for healthcare professionals fron the American Heart Association. Writing Group. Circulation 1995;91:580-615.Fletcher GF, Balady G, Froelicher VF, Hartley LH, Haskell WL, Pollock ML).

Effects of Physical Activity on Disability and Functional Limitation

Old women are less physically active when compared to men in the same age range. Physical inactivity can be regarded as a risk factor for the development of functional limitation. Brown and coll. have shown how old women with pre existing functional limitation are less physically active when compared to women without disability (physical activity among adults > or= 50 yr with or without disabilities; BRFSS 2001; Med Sci Sports Exerc.2005;37:620-629.Brown DR,Yore MM, Ham SA, Macera CA.). However, evidence about physical activity in old women is still largely insufficient. Furthermore, the American College of Sport Medicine recommendations are often very difficult to implement in the clinical setting of the elderly because of the great physiological and pathological variability that characterize such a population. In a longitudinal study physical inactivity, as assessed by self report, was shown to strongly associate to pre existing functional limitation, in community-dwelling women, aged 70-79 years. One of our goals should, therefore, be to implement physical activity programs in the elderly with disability and to appropriately modify the type, intensity and frequency of exercise on the basis of the underlying functional limitations and chronic diseases (Physycal Activity by presence and type of functional deficits in older women: the Women's Healt and Aging Studies; J of Gerontology 2006, vol 61, no 11, 1171-1176, Gerald J.Jerome, Thomas A.Glass, Micelle Miele, Qian-Li Xue, Ross E.Andersen, Linda P.Field).

A number of studies have shown that physical activity can prevent, or at least decrease, functional limitation and disability even in old women.

The Lifestyle Interventions and Indipendence for Elders Pilot (LIFE P) Study showed that increasing physical activity in the elderly decreases functional limitation and improves performance (especially leg performance), thus allowing a higher degree of autonomy (A little exercise, Journal of Gerontology, 2006 Vol61A,no 11, 1154-1156, Luigi Ferrucci and Eleanor M Simonsick).. Physical activity not only improves quality of life and promotes well-being, but it can substantially decrease the economic burden on our health care systems.

Chronic diseases represent a major cause of disability and functional decline among the elderly (Benefits of exercise for community dwelling older adults;Arch Phys Med Rehabil Vol 85, Suppl 3, July 2004.Jonathan F.Bean, MD, MS,Ariona Vora, MD, Walter R.Frontera, MD). The most common chronic diseases in this population are: osteoarthritis, cardiovascular disease, diabetes, lung diseases and stroke. As many as 60 % of women and 50 % of men over 70 suffer from osteoarthritis, while cardiovascular disease is present in 40% and 31% of women and men over 65, respectively. Stroke, diabetes and lung diseases are present in more than 10 % of the people over 65. Osteoporosis represents another extremely frequent condition in the elderly: its prevalence is more than tripled in men and women over 85, compared to the population in the 65–74 age range. It is largely acknowledged that such diseases are a major cause of disability, hospitalization and death among the elderly. The available evidence suggests that physical activity can improve autonomy and decrease the degree of functional decline in patients with chronic diseases. Exercise has shown to decrease pain and disability in patients with osteoarthritis, and is therefore recommended by the American Geriatrics Society (American Geriatrics Society Panel on Exercise and Osteoarthritis pain: consensus practice recommendations. Supplement to the AGS Clinical Practice Guidelines on the management of chronic pain in older adults; J Am Geriatr Soc 2001;49:808-23). Furthermore, two RCTs have shown that brist walking can improve muscular strength and resistance in elderly suffering from osteoarthritis (Progressive resistence stength training for physical disability in older people, The Cochrane Library, 2003. Latham N, Anderson CS, Bennett D, Stretton C.) (Effectiveness of exercise therapy in patients with osteoarthritis of the tip or knee: a systematic review of randomized clinical trials. Arthritis Rheum 1999;42: 1361-9. Van Baar ME, Assendelft WJ, Dekker J, Oostendorp RA, Bijlsma JW).

Table 2.

Health Issue	Benefits of Physical Activity
Cardiovascular Healt	Improves myocardial performance Increases peak diastolic filling Increases heart muscle contractility Reduce premature ventricular contraction Improves blood lipid profile Increases aerobic capacity Reduces systolic blood pressure Improves diastolic blood pressure Improves endurance Improves muscle capillary blood flow
Body Composition	Decreases abdominal adipose tissue Increases muscle mass
Metabolism	Increases total energy expenditure Improves protein synthesis rate and amino acid uptake Into the skeletal muscle Reduce very-low and low-density lipoproteins Reduce triglycerides Increases high-density lipoproteins Increase glucose-tolerance
Bone Healt	Slows decline in bone mineral density Increases total body calcium
Psychological Well-Being	Improves perceived well-being and happiness Decreases levels of stress-related hormones Improves attention span Improves cognitive processing speed Increases slow wave and rapid eye movement sleep
Muscle Weakness and Functional Capacity	Reduces risk of musculoskeletal disability Improves strength and flexibility Reduces risk of falls Improves dynamic balance Improves physical functional performance

Physical activity programs and behaviour counselling in older adults populations .Medicine and Science in sports and exercise 2004 M Ealine Cress, David M. Buchner, Thomas Prohaska, James Rimmel, Marybeth Brown, Carol Macera, Loretta DePietro, Wojtek Chodzko-Zajko.

Miller and coll. have shown that, among the elderly with osteoarthritis, those who where more active physically had a slower progression of functional limitation, during a follow-up period of 6 years (data adjusted for age, gender, comorbidity and previous functional capacity) (Physical activity, fubctional limitations, and disability in older adults. J Am Geriatr Soc 2000;48:1264-72. Miller ME, Rejeski WJ, Reboussin BA, Ten Have TR, Ettinger WH).

However, evidence about the beneficial effects of physical activity in preventing and minimizing disability is still lacking. In fact, most studies have overlooked disability as an outcome. On the other hand, data from the studies that took it into account are inconsistent, a beneficial effect having being detected only in 35 % of such studies. Among the RCTs that have confirmed a beneficial effects of physical activity on disability, only 3 have studied elderly patients with osteoarthritis while 3 other RCTs have studied both community dwelling and institutionalized patients with functional limitation. The Fitness Arthritis and Seniors Trial (FAST) has studied more than 400 subjects, over 60, with a radiological diagnosis of osteoarthritis, pain and limitations in the daily activities; subjects were randomized to a programme of physical activity (including aerobic and resistance exercise) or to an educational intervention. The FAST was the only RCT that could show a strong association between physical activity and disability in patients with osteoarthritis: after 18 months the active arm of the study showed a greater improvement in ADL scores when compared to the educational intervention arm (A Randomized trial comparing aerobic exercise and resistance exercise with a healt education program in older adults with knee osteoarthritis and seniors trial. JAMA 1997;277:25-31. Ettinger WH, Burns R, Messier SP et al).

Being the evidence from RCTs insufficient, we must rely on data from observational studies when considering the beneficial effects of exercise on disability in subjects with osteoarthritis.

Two prospective studies, including 5151 and 1321 elderly respectively and with a follow-up of 2 and 3 years respectively, have shown that physically active subjects develop lower degrees of disability (as assessed by ADL) when compared to the inactive.

The Established Populations of Epidemiological Studies of the Elderly (EPESE) have shown that the most active subjects develop less disability in their whole life span, when compared to the inactive. It is well acknowledged how exercise, especially brist walking, can improve strength, aerobic capacity and function. However, it is not as clear if exercise can decrease the degree of pre existing disability. Often the power of exercise studies is impaired by the short follow-up period: in fact, a trial with a 18 month follow-up showed that exercise could actually improve pre existing disability. Unfortunately, most of the studies have follow-up periods of 8-12 weeks. Other common limitations of the studies dealing with physical activity are the exclusion of subjects with functional impairment and the assessment of data about exercise type and intensity through self-reports. Furthermore, it is often difficult to compare data from different trials, as different definitions, or even no definitions, of exercise and physical activity are provided. In order to be able to compare and pool data in the literature, it is fundamental to establish definitions that are accepted by all the Authors. Understanding which features of exercise are the most important (type, intensity, duration, frequency) must be regarded as a key step of such process (Does Late-Life Physical Activity or Exercise Prevent or Minimize Disablement? Am J Prev Med 2003;25:129-136. Julie J. Keysor PhD,PT). Strong evidence is available about the benefits of physical activity in the elderly with chronic cardiovascular disease. Old women with coronary artery disease (CAD) have a decreased aerobic capacity (as assessed by aerobic peak power: VO2 peak), a decreased muscular strength and a lower quality of life (QOL). A study has compared the effects of aerobic exercise alone and aerobic exercise combined with strength training (COMT) on VO2 peak, total distance on 6 minute walking test, muscular strength (measured at upper and lower limbs), in 18 women, aged 60-80 years, with known CAD. Aerobic exercise and strength training improved VO2 peak, total distance walked in 6 minutes, limb muscular strength and QOL, but upper limb strength and QOL still improved after 8 weeks of COMT while they did not improve further with aerobic exercise alone. The best results have been observed in old women with CAD who underwent a program of cardiologic rehabilitation including both aerobic exercise and strength training. This study confirmed that physical activity can improve aerobic capacity, muscular strength and QOL. However, these results should be interpreted carefully, as the study dataset was extremely small (Exercise training improves overall physical fitness and quality of life in older women with coronary artery disease, CHEST 2004; 126:1026-1031; Chihya Hung, Bill Daub, Bill Black, Robert Welsh, Arthur Quinney and Mark Haykowsky).

Heart failure (HF), often characterized by impaired diastolic function, is commonly seen among the elderly: in a study 32 women, suffering from diastolic HF, where randomized to a program of moderate intensity home physical activity, of the duration of 12 weeks, or to an educational program.

The 6-minute-walk-test performance, the QOL (as assessed by the Living With Heart Failure Questionnaire) and depression (as assessed by the Geriatric Depression Scale) all improved in the physical activity arm. In conclusion, in old women with HF, the implementation of an educational intervention, combined with a program of mild physical activity at home, would be a realistic means of improving functional capacity and QOL. It must be said, however, that studies that confirm the utility of such a strategy in the long period are still lacking (Home-based exercise improves functional performance and quality of lie in women with diastolic heart failure; Heart Lung 2004 Jul-Aug;33:210-8. Gary RA, Sueta CA, Dougherty M, Rosemberg B, Cheek D, Preisser J, Neelon V, McMurray R).

In a RCT, we evaluated the effects of a program of mild physical activity in the elderly. Four hundred thirty eight patients were enrolled and randomized to the physical activity arm or to the control group. The type and intensity of physical activity was assessed through self-report questionnaires. Pharmacotherapy, referral to the health-care system, energy expenditure, deambulation , QOL and subjective perception of the quality of the ongoing program were the main outcomes we evaluated. We observed no significant modification in the functional capacity of the control group, while we observed a mild improvement of walking distance, of balance, of QOL and a decrease in health-care system referrals in the active group (Invecchiare in salute, I risultati di una Ricerca-Intervento sull'efficacia dei corsi di ginnastica per anziani a Torino, Regione Piemonte, 2004).

Effects of Physical Activity on Survival and Mortality

Motor skills result from the complex interaction of the central nervous system (cerebellum, basal ganglia, pre-frontal, parietal and primary cortical motor areas), the peripheral nervous system (motor neurons) and the skeletal muscles.

A longitudinal observational study, that evaluated the correlation between motor function and mortality, showed that motor performance and muscular strength worsen with ageing. Furthermore, such changes were associated with an excess in mortality rates. Besides the para-physiological, age-correlated changes, there is a number of pathological conditions (e.g. Parkinson disease, stroke, degenerative diseases) that affect the nervous system and that can cause alterations in the motor skills. Such diseases could explain some of the excess in mortality rates observed in individuals with motor limitation. The Rush Memory and Aging Project evaluated the effects of physical activity in 800 old subjects, free from cognitive impairment: motor skills and muscular strength of the limbs and of respiratory muscles were assessed both *in vivo* and *post-mortem*. The study showed that mortality is reduced by 10% *per* year by physical activity. Mortality was reduced by as much as 30% when active subjects are compared to the subjects with most evident motor limitation (Change in Motor Function and Risk of Mortality in Older Persons;American Geriatrics Society,gen 2007, 55:11-19,Aron S. Buchman, Robert S. Wilson, Patricia A.Boyle, Julia L. Bienias, David A.Bennet). Muscular strength and the degree of changes in strength are strongly associated to total mortality, with no differences between genders. A longitudinal study evaluated the effects of body composition changes on performance status, in 74 women and 66 men, over 65, over a follow-up of 3 years. It was observed that, even without any change in body weight, lean mass decreases steadily, while fat mass (especially abdominal fat) increases; a negative correlation was shown between abdominal fat burden, lean mass reduction and reported duration, frequency and intensity of physical activity. Furthermore, steady physical activity is believed to reduce abdominal fat mass, while helping to maintain lean mass (A 3-years longitudinal study on body composition changes in the elderly; role of physical exercise. Clin Nurt 2006Aug; 25: 573-80. Raguso CA, Kyle U, Kossovsky MP, Roynette C, Paoloni-Giacobino A, Hans D, Genton L, Pichard C).

A study that enrolled 7023 subjects, of both sexes, aged 20-79 years, showed a greater mortality in the inactive subjects and an improved survival in those who engaged in mild physical activity programs, independent of gender and age (Changes in Leisure-time Physical Activity and Risk of Death: an observational study of 7000 Men and Women, American Journal of Epidemiology 2003, 158,639, Peter Schnohr, Henrik Scharling, and Jan Skov Jensen).

Data from a study, that evaluated the effects of low intensity physical activity, like walking, in 707 retired males without functional limitation, aged 61-81 years, are shown in Table 3.

Table 3.

	Miles/day	Mortality rate(%)
All-causes (n. 208)	0.0-0.9	40.5
	1.0-2.0	27.4
	2.1-8.0	23.8
CHD/stroke (n.52)	0.0-0.9	6.2
	1.0-2.0	5.5
	2.1-8.0	2.3
Cancer (n. 68)	0.0-0.9	12.8
	1.0-2.0	9.4
	2.1-8.0	5.6

Effects of Walking on Mortality Among non smoking retired men Ami A Hakim MS, Elen Petrovitch MD, Cecil M Burchfiel PhD, G. Webster Ross MD, Beatriz L. Rodriguez MD PhD, Lon R White MD, Katsuhico Yano MD, David Curb MD, and Robert D Abbott MD. New England Journal of Medicine 338, 94-99, 8 january 1998).

The study showed a correlation between the distance walked in a day and total cause mortality, after a follow-up of 12 years (Effects of Walking on Mortality Among non smoking retired men Ami A Hakim MS, Elen Petrovitch MD, Cecil M Burchfiel PhD, G. Webster Ross MD, Beatriz L. Rodriguez MD PhD, Lon R White MD, Katsuhico Yano MD, David Curb MD, and Robert D Abbott MD. New England Journal of Medicine 338, 94-99, 8 january 1998).

Evidence supporting the benefits of physical activity in old subjects with chronic cardiovascular disease is strong. Aerobic physical activity enhances energy expenditure and improves cardiovascular performance, which implies a lower incidence of obesity and a decrease in total cardiovascular risk burden. In the elderly, the correlation between the degree of physical activity and cardiovascular fitness is particularly strong: intense cardiovascular fitness prevents the development of cardiovascular disease, while a high energetic expenditure helps in the regulation of body weight and composition.

It is known that energy expenditure and aerobic capacity decrease with aging, by about 12-30%. Furthermore, the level of physical activity has been estimated to be approximately one third in older subjects, when compared to the young. Two studies have evaluated the correlation between cardiovascular fitness and energy expenditure in women in the 66-82 age range: there was a significant association between moderate-intense physical activity and cardiovascular fitness, while no data are available about mild intensity physical activity. According to a metanalysis, however, cardiovascular risk is decreased more consistently by aerobic physical activity than by mild non-aerobic training (Impact of cardiovascular fitness and physical activity level on health outcomes in older persons, Mechanisms of ageing and development, 2003, 259-267. Isabelle J Dionne, Philip A Ades, Eric T Poehlman).

Hypertension, CAD and HF represent the second cause of chronic disability and the leading cause of death, in the elderly. A metanalysis and 2 reviews have shown that moderate intensity physical activity, in women, is associated with a 2% (i.e. 11 mmHg) and a 1% (i.e. 8 mmHg) reduction in systolic and diastolic blood pressure (BP) respectively, thus favouring a regression of left ventricular hypertrophy. A combined program of aerobic exercise and resistance training seems to be even more effective in lowering systolic and diastolic BP (2 and 4% reductions, respectively). Furthermore, the benefits of physical activity on BP seems to be independent of age (Progressive Resistance exercise and resting blood pressure: a meta-analysis of randomized controlled trials. Hypertension 2000;35:838-43. Kelley GA,Kelley KS). A metanalysis compared the effects of physical activity alone or combined with a cardiologic rehabilitation program, in patients with a previous myocardial infarction: mortality was reduced by 31 and 26% by exercise alone and by the combined intervention, respectively; the cardiologic rehabilitation program showed the potential for lowering low density lipoprotein (LDL) cholesterol levels as well. However, because of the low numerosity of the dataset, it is not possible to draw conclusions about the superiority of any of 2 the intervention protocols (Exercise-based rehabilitation for coronary heart disease. Cochrane Database Syst Rev 2001;CD 001800.Jolliffe JA,Rees K, Taylor RS, Thompson D,Oldridge N, Ebrahim S.).

Physical activity not only acts on a number of the pathological mechanisms of HF (e.g. myopathy, rhythm abnormalities and cytokine expression), but it relieves the symptoms and improves resistance capacity, in patients with HF (exercise training as a therapy for chronic heart failure: can older people benefit? J Am Geriatr Soc 2003;51:699-709. Witham MD, Struthers AD, McMurdo ME). Data on long term effects of physical activity on morbidity and mortality, in such patients, are still lacking. Furthermore, the role of walking, as compared to intense physical training, in the prevention of cardiovascular disease is controversial. This is especially true about women: more than 40 epidemiological studies have evaluated the correlation between coronary heart disease and physical activity, but very few such studies included women. However, available data suggest that benefits of physical activity are similar in males and females, with a relative risk reduction of 30-50% in both genders. In a study that enrolled 72488 women, aged 40-65 years, without a previous diagnosis of cardiovascular disease, walking and intense physical training were associated with a similar reduction (30-40%) in the incidence of new coronary events (defined as coronary death or nonfatal myocardial infarction), during a follow-up period of 8 years. Among physically active women, there was a lower prevalence of diabetic, hypertensive, dyslipidemic and smoking subjects. In this study the degree of physical activity was unrelated to age, family history of coronary events or diet fat intake. In conclusion, in this study, physical activity showed an inverse correlation with the risk of new coronary events in women, regardless of body weight, smoking and family history (A Prospective Study of walking is compared with vigorous exercise in the prevention of coronary heart disease in women; The New England Journal of Medicine, 26 august 1999, Manson E., Frank B., Janet W., Rich-Edwards, Graham A.Colditz, Meir J. Stampfer,Walter C.Willet, Frank E. Speizer, Charles H.Hennekens). Two recent studies have shown that walking, approximately 4 hours *per* week, was effective in substantially reducing cardiovascular risk in old women and men. However, it is not clear if benefits from physical activity can be affected by environmental and genetic variability, in different populations. Among the 73743 women, in post-menopausal age, enrolled in the Women's Health Initiative, those walking 30 minutes 5 times *per* week ($\geq$ 2.5 hours *per* week) experienced a 30% reduction in the risk for cardiovascular events, after a median follow-up of 3.2 years. A similar risk reduction was seen in women training more intensely. Among women over 65, those walking more than 4 hours *per* week had a substantial reduction in the risk of hospitalization, when compared to women walking less than 1 hour *per* week (Does walking decrease the risk of cardiovascular disease hospitalizations and death in olders adults? J Am Geriatr Soc 1996;44:113-120. La Croix AZ, Leveille SG, Hecht JA, Grothaus LC, Wagner EH).

In a study, that enrolled 73743 post-menopausal women, aged 50-59 years the women that were not overweight, did not smoke, followed a balanced diet and exercised 30-60 minutes, at moderate-high intensity, on a daily basis, showed a reduction in the relative risk of new cardiovascular events of approximately 80 %, after a follow-up period of 5.9 years. However, a selection bias was present in this study, as the enrolled subjects were at low risk for coronary events; furthermore results were not adjusted for the use of medications, such as antihypertensive therapy or hormonal replacement therapy (Primary Prevention of Coronary Heart Disease in women througth diet and lifestyle Meir J Stampfer M.D., Frank B HU M.D., Joanne Manson M.D., Eric B Rimm, SC.D., and Walter C Willet M.D.,New England Journal of Medicine 2000, 343:16-22).

A number of mechanisms may contribute to the reduction in cardiovascular mortality and morbidity in the physically active subjects. Thirty minutes of moderate intensity exercise, on a daily basis, have been shown to substantially reduce cardiovascular risk, with little effect on body weight; longer periods of physical activity are, in fact, required in order to achieve a substantial reduction in body weight: a significant reduction in adiposity was observed in menopausal women, previously overweight and inactive, after one year moderate intensity training (45 minutes, 5 times per week), despite no substantial changes in the diet. (Effect of exercise on total intra-abdominal body fat in postmenopausal women: a randomized rail. JAMA 2003, 289:323-330. Irwin ML, Yasui Y, Ulrich CM, Bowen D, Rudolph RE, Schwartz RS, Yukawa M, Aiello E, Potter JD, McTiernam A). On the other hand, according to the available data, it is possible to hypothesize that 30 minutes of moderate intensity training *per* day, together with a moderate reduction in caloric intake can help achieve a similar weight reduction. Training 30 minutes *per* day has also shown to be effective in reducing blood pressure and improve lipid profile and insulin-sensitivity, thus reducing cardiovascular burden. A reduction in fibrinogen and C reactive protein levels has also been described, suggesting a regulatory action of physical activity on inflammation and hemostasis. However this relationship has been studied only in males and needs to be further investigated (Physical activity and the prevention of cardiovascular disease. Curr Atheroscler. Rep 5 2003; 299-299-307. Bassuk SS, Manson JE).

In a prospective study that followed, for 24 years, 116564 women, aged 30-55 years, without known cardiovascular disease or neoplasm, 10282 deaths were observed : 2370 (23%) subjects died of a cardiovascular cause, 5223 (50,8%) subjects died of cancer and 2689 (26.2%) subjects died of other causes (Table 4).

Table 4.

Physical activity (hour/week)			
BMI	>=3.5	1.0-3.4	<1.0
All death			
<25	1.00	1.18 (1.09-1.29)	1.55(1.42-1.70)
25-29.9	1.28 (1.12-1.46)	1.33(1.20-1.47)	1.64(1.46-1.83)
>=30	1.91(1.60-2.30)	2.05(1.82-2.30)	2.42(2.14-2.73)
CV death			
<25	1.00	1.51(1.22-1.87)	1.89(1.51-2.37)
25-29.9	1.58(1.15-2.16)	2.06(1.62-2.60)	2.52(1.96-3.25)
>=30	2.87(1.94-4.25)	4.26(3.33-5.44)	4.73(3.68-6.09)
Cancer			
<25	1.00	1.09(0.98-1.22)	1.32(1.17-1.50)
25-29.9	1.22 (1.02-1.45)	1.20(1.05-1.38)	1.39(1.19-1.62)
>=30	1.57(1.21-2-03)	1.44(1.21-1.71)	1.68(1.40-2.01)

Adiposity as Compared with Physical Activity in Predicting Mortality among Women, New England Journal of Medicine 351, 23 december 2004 Frank B. Hu, M.D., Walter C. Willett, M.D., Tricia Li, M.D., Meir J. Stampfer, M.D.,Graham A. Colditz, M.D., and JoAnn E. Manson, M.D).

In this dataset overweight was asssociated with a substantially higher mortality; physical activity proved to be ineffective in reducing the risk excess associated with obesity, while benefits were observed across all the degrees of overweight (Adiposity as Compared with Physical Activity in Predicting Mortality among Women, New England Journal of Medicine 351, 23 december 2004 Frank B. Hu, M.D., Walter C. Willett, M.D., Tricia Li, M.D., Meir J. Stampfer, M.D.,Graham A. Colditz, M.D., and JoAnn E. Manson, M.D).

Paradoxically, an inverse correlation was found between obesity and mortality in subjects suffering from heart failure, coronary heart disease requiring interventional management or end-stage renal failure. In 6876 subjects (mean age 55 years) the mortality rate of the obese subjects was 33% lower than the mortality rate of subjects in the normal weight range, with a 3% gain in survival for each BMI unit. The protective effect of overweight could be partly explained by the larger amount of muscles and by the larger diameter of coronary arteries that characterize overweight subjects. However the relationship between fitness, obesity and mortality is complex, thus requiring further studies and research (Body mass, Fitness and

Survival in Veteran Patients: Another Obesità Paradox? The American Journal of Medicine 2007, 120,518-524, Paul McAuley, Jonathan Myers, Joshua Abella, Victor Froelicher).

A longitudinal study evaluated the effects of lifestyle modifications on the incidence of metabolic syndrome in men aged 60-79 years, without cardiovascular disease or diabetes, during a follow-up period of 3 years. Overweight, obesity, physical inactivity, smoking and high carbohydrate intake are all well known risk factors for the development of the metabolic syndrome; even among the elderly, the abolition of such risk factors results in a dramatic fall in the incidence of the syndrome, and should therefore be considered as a fundamental primary prevention measure (Modifiable Lifestyle Factors and the Metabolic Syndrom in Older Men: Effects of Lifestyle Changes, Journal of the American Geriatrics Society, vol 54, issue 12, december 2006, 1909-1914S Goya Wannamethee, A Gerald Shaker, Peter H Whincup).

Diabetes is an important cause of mortality and morbidity in the elderly; its prevalence has been increasing dramatically in the past two decades. Regular physical activity has been shown effective in reducing cardiovascular complications and mortality in subjects with diabetes (Relationship of walking to mortalità among US adults with diabetes. Arch Int Med 2003;163:1440-7. Gregg EW, Gerzoff RB, Caspersen CJ, Williamson DF, Narayan KM); furthermore, moderate exercise is effective in preventing the development of type 2 diabetes. Baule et al. have showed that physical activity can increase insulin-sensitivity, decrease HbA1c levels, improve lipid profile and decrease blood pressure, thus reducing the cardiovascular burden and the risk for complications in patients with diabetes. Exercise must therefore be considered a fundamental component of preventive strategies in these patients (Effect of exercise on glycemic control and body mass in type 2 diabetes mellitus: a meta-analysis of controlled clinical trias;JAMA 2001 286:1218-27.Boule NG, Haddad E, Kenny GP, Wells GA, Sigal RJ). However, data about exercise in patients over 60 are lacking, only 3 of the 14 revised studies having enrolled subjects over 60. It would be important to evaluate the effects of training in the steadily growing population of the elderly with diabetes, through a RCT.

It must also be remembered that many elderly with diabetes have serious functional limitation and disability, thus making intense physical activity an unrealistic therapeutic strategy (Diabetes and physical disability among older US adults. Diabetes Care 2000; 23:1272-7. Gregg EW, Beckls GL, Williamson DF, Leveille SG, Langlois JA, Engelgau MM et al). A few studies have evaluated the effects of walking in old diabetic subjects with disability: those walking more than 1 mile *per* day experienced a significant decrease in all-cause mortality. Even though the protective effects of walking extend to old subjects without diabetes, they appear to be stronger in the diabetics. A study that enrolled 1664 subjects, aged 50-90 years, with type 2 diabetes have evaluated the effects of walking on mortality in both subjects with and without diabetes. Approximately half of the enrolled subjects were women, among them 71% was hypertensive and 32% had known cardiovascular disease. During the 10-year follow-up 564 subjects died from both cardiovascular and non-cardiovascular causes; however all-cause mortality was reduced by almost 50% in subjects with diabetes that walked at least 1 mile *per* day. A reduction in cardiovascular mortality was also observed in adults without diabetes that walked more than 1 mile *per* day, but there were no significant differences in cardiovascular mortality, or in mortality from other causes, among adults with and without diabetes who walked 1 mile *per* day. Age, male gender, smoking and history of cardiovascular disease are all independent predictors of mortality, while training more than 3 times *per* week has shown to protect from death from coronary artery disease. In this study, the benefits of walking were consistent across genders (Walking decreased risk of cardiovascular disease mortality in older adults with diabetes. Journal of Clinical Epidemiology 60 2007 309-317. Tyler C. Smith, Deborah L. Wingard, Besa Smith, Donna Kritz-Silvestein, Elizabeth Barrett-Connor). After adjusting results for sex, gender, BMI, smoking, alcohol consumption, exercise, blood pressure, history of cardiovascular disease the analysis showed that walking more than 1 mile *per* day provided a strong protection against all-cause mortality in the elderly with diabetes. A metanalysis showed no significant interaction between gender and diabetes (Explaining the sex difference in coronary heart disease mortality among patients with tipe 2 diabetes mellitus: a meta-analysis. Arch Intern Med 2002; 162: 1737-45. Kanaya AM, Grady D, Barret-Connor E). It is likely that the stronger protective effects of walking seen in the subjects with diabetes, compared to subjects without diabetes, depend on the higher prevalence of overweight, obesity, hypertension, dyslipidaemia and physical inactivity in such patients. Exercise, in fact, modifies cardiovascular burden by acting on these risk factors. The evidence that even mild physical activity can result in a reduction in mortality allows to tailor exercise programs to the population of the elderly with diabetes, as a part of interventions aiming to improve quality of life and prevent cardiovascular complications.

PHYSICAL ACTIVITY AND CHRONIC DISEASES

Exercise recommendations, tailored to some common chronic diseases are shown in Table 5.

Amongst lung disorders, obstructive diseases (chronic bronchitis, emphysema and asthma) have a prevalence as high as 11% in adults over 70. Evidence from metanalyses or reviews as to the effects of physical activity in subjects with chronic obstructive pulmonary disease (COPD) is lacking. However, in a few studies an improvement in dyspnoea and functional capacity (as assessed by the 6 minute walking test) was observed, in such patients (power of outcomes measurements to detect clinically significant changes in pulmonary rehabilitation of patients with COPD. Chest 2002; 121:1092-8.De Torres JP, Pinto-Plota V, Ingenito E et al).

Eleven percent of the subjects over 70 are affected by chronic obstructive pulmonary disease (COPD) (chronic bronchitis, emphysema and asthma). High level evidence, from metanalysis or reviews, about the effects of physical activity in subjects with COPD is lacking; however, in a few studies an improvement in dyspnoea and functional capacity (as assessed by the 6 minute walking test) was observed, in such patients (power of outcomes measurements to detect clinically significant changes in pulmonary rehabilitation of patients with COPD. Chest 2002; 121:1092-8.De Torres JP, Pinto-Plota V, Ingenito E et al).

A number of RCTs and metanalysis have shown that exercise can increase bone and muscular mass, thus reducing the risk of osteoporosis and fractures: the incidence of fractures was reduced by as much as 37% by walking, strength and balance exercise (Falls prevention over 2 years: a randomized controlled trial in women 80 years and older. Age Ageing 1999;28: 513-8. Compobell AJ, Robertson MC, Gordner MM, Norton RN, Buchner DM).

Among women, isometric exercise not only improves glycaemia, lipid profile and blood pressure, but also greatly enhances skeletal muscles function; we can, thus, speculate that physical activity is even more effective in reducing the risk of fractures in women, as compared with men. It is not known which type of physical activity has the most beneficial effects in preventing osteoporosis and its complications, but it can be hypothesized that a combination of the different types can act synergistically to improve bone mass and muscular function.

Table 5. Recommendations for Independent Exercise, by Medical Condition

Conditions	Recommendation
Osteoarthritis, Cardiovascular Disease,Diabetes	PRT 2–3 times weekly at 13–17 on the Borg Scale 2–3 sets of 8–10 repetitions Greater strength gains will be achieved at higher Borg Scale ratings Aerobic training Examples: walking, biking, aquatic exercise 2–3 times weekly Progress up to 30–40min 11–13 on the Borg Scale
Respiratory Disease	Train both upper and lower extremities separately at 60% exercise-tested maximal work capacity, which is roughly equivalent to 11–13 on the Borg Scale Upper-body exercises include arm ergometry, canoeing, swimming, low-resistance high repetition weight lifting Lower-body exercises include walking, stationary bicycling, stair climbing Perform exercise 3–5 times weekly progressing to 30–60min/session Self-monitor dyspnea Increase intensity every 5th session as tolerated Theoretical benefits of PRT at higher intensities are yet to be shown
Stroke	PRT 2–3 times weekly at 13–17 on the Borg Scale 2–3 sets of 8–10 repetitions Greater strength gains will be achieved at higher Borg Scale ratings Aerobic training Treadmill walking at normal gait speed or slightly faster More impaired subjects may benefit from supported treadmill walking 2–3 times weekly Progress to 30–40min 11–13 on the Borg Scale Task-specific training Perform functional tasks such as rising from chair, climbing stairs, squatting Progress to 2–3 sets of 8–10 repetitions

Table 5. (Continued).

Conditions	Recommendation
Osteoporosis	PRT 2–3 times weekly at 13–17 on the Borg Scale 2–3 sets of 8–10 repetitions Note greater strength gains will be achieved at higher Borg Scale ratings Specific attention to spinal extensors is important Aerobic exercise Only strenuous aerobic exercise, including combinations of fast walking, stair climbing, jogging, or calisthenics have been shown to be beneficial
Falls, Poor balance, and Mobility Problems	PRT 2–3 times weekly at 13–17 on the Borg Scale 2–3 sets of 8–10 repetitions Note greater strength gains will be achieved at higher Borg Scale ratings Aerobic training Examples: walking, biking, aquatic exercise 2–3 times weekly Progress to 30–40min 11–13 on the Borg Scale Dynamic exercises Tai Chi High-velocity training: exercises with concentric component performed as quickly as possible to augment muscle power Examples: repeated performance of leg exercises on exercise machines or common functional tasks such as chair rise or climbing a step.

NOTE. All recommendations assume that the patient has successfully passed appropriate screening and monitoring procedures to assess safety for independent exercise. Physical activity programs and behaviour counselling in older adults populations. Medicine and Science in sports and exercise 2004 Physical activity programs and behaviour counselling in older adults populations. Medicine and Science in sports and exercise 2004 Benefits of exercise for community dwelling older adults;Arch Phys Med Rehabil Vol 85, Suppl 3, July 2004.Jonathan f. bean, MD, MS,Ariona Vora, MD, Walter R.Frontera, MD.

Physical Activity and Cognition

Dementia is an age-related disease and its prevalence increases steadily with aging. A few trials have evaluated the effects of physical activity on cognitive decline and dementia. However, the evidence here revised is mainly supported by observational studies while data from RCTs are still insuffcient (Physical activity and cognition in old age; Current Opinion in Psychiatry 2006;19:190-193; Nicola T. Lavtenschloger and Osvaldo P.Almeida). An observational study followed 5925 old women for 6-8 years in order to compare the degree of cognitive decline among physically active and inactive subjects; the Nurses Health Study enrolled 19000 women, aged 70-81 years, with a follow-up of 8-15 years. These studies showed that exercise, even walking, was associated with a significantly lower degree of cognitive decline and that physically active subjects had a better cognitive performance. In a review, exercise not only reduced the risk of developing Alzheimer disease, but even improved cognition in subjects with pre-existing cognitive impairment or dementia (the effects of exercise training on elderly persons withcognitive impairment and dementia;a meta-analysis;Arch Phys Med Rehabil 2004;85:1694-1704.Heyn P, Abrev BC, Ottenbacher Kj).

A study on women aged 70-81 years showed that intense exercise is associated with a higher cognitive performance, as assessed by 6 tests addressing memory, attention and language skills. Furthermore in this study physically active women had a 20% lower risk of cognitive decline, when compared to sedentary women (Physical activity, includine walking, and cognitive function in older women. JAMA 2004 sep 22;292:1454-61. Weuve J, Kang JH, Manson JE, Breteler MM, Ware JH, Grodstein F).

Dissemination of the benefits of physical activity has proven ineffective in promoting the adherence of the elderly to exercise programs: it is fundamental to identify and abolish the barriers that prevent radical changes in the lifestyle of the elderly.

Table 6. Common Barriers to Exercise in Older Adults

Barrier	Approach
Self-efficacy	Begin slowly with exercises that are easily accomplished; advance gradually; provide frequent encouragement.
Attitude	Promote positive personal benefits of exercise; identify enjoyable activities.
Discomfort	Vary intensity and range of exercise; employ crosstraining; start slowly; avoid overdoing.
Poor balance/ataxia	Assistive devices can increase safety as well as increase exercise intensity.
Fear of injury	Balance and strength training initially; use of appropriate clothing, equipment, and supervision; start slowly.
Habit	Incorporate into daily routine; repeat encouragement; promote active lifestyle.*
Subjective norms	Identify and recruit influential others; education of patient and influential family/friends.
Fixed income	Walking and other simple exercises; use of household items; promote active lifestyle.
Environmental factors (e.g., inclement weather)	Walk in the mall; use senior centers; promote active lifestyle.
Cognitive decline	Incorporate into daily routine; keep exercises simple.
Illness/fatigue	Use a range of exercises/intensities that patients can match to their varying energy level.

*—Examples of an active lifestyle include using a golf pull cart while golfing, using a push mower, participating in activities such as stand and cast fishing or gardening, and taking the stairs. Promoting and Prescribing Exercise for the Elderly;American Family Physician february 1, 2002, Robert J Nied, Barry Franklin.

The aim should be to promote a more active lifestyle, that should then be maintained over the whole life span, in the elderly; in order to obtain good adherence rates it is probably necessary to offer the elderly mild exercise programs. The cognitive-behavioural approach is thought to be fundamental in promoting physical activity and exercise among adults, however there are few data on the analysis of the cognitive processes related to physical activity and about disability.

Table 7. Selected content of physical activity programs for older adults from major organizations and institutions

Resource	Endurance	Strength	Flexibility/Range of Motion	Balance	Programming	Special Conditions	Appropriate audience
ACSM Fitness Book 3rd Edition	Walking and large muscle groups.	13 exercises, free weights and body weight.	21 exercises	Limited coverage	Lifestyle Safety Programming Evaluation	Limited coverage	Exercise participant (middle and young-old ages).
ACSM Resource Manual: 4th Edition	Types of fitness, goal setting, developing exercise sessions, progression and maintenance.	Precautions, patients with cardiovascular disease recommendations.	Techniques for static stretching and proprioceptive neuromuscular facilitation; 23 exercises illustrated	Limited specific coverage	Injuries: risks, prevention and care.	Patients with cardiovascular diseases, diabetes, hypertension, peripheral arterial disease, osteoporosis, chronic lung disease.	Professional wanting underlying scientific basis for recommendations.
American Council on Exercise: Exercise for Older Adults Book	Techniques in group exercise.	7 exercises, free weights. 6 exercises, elastic bands.	11 exercises	3 exercises	Lifestyle Safety Programming Group-based Leadership	Major chronic conditions, medications	Lay or professional Exercise leaders.
Exercise: A guide from the National Institute on Aging Book/ Video	Lifestyle activities.	12 exercises, free weights and body weight.	12 exercises	6 exercises	Lifestyle Safety Programming Individual Evaluation	Limited coverage	Older adult participant.
Exercise for Frail Elders	10 seated	14 exercises, elastic, free and Velcro® strapped on weights	24 exercises	0	Safety Programming Group-based	Comprehensive section on Chronic conditions	Lay or professional Exercise leader

Programming included strategies for integrating balance, strength and flexibility into programs or lifestyle activities, sample schedules with days of the week for strength, endurance and flexibility training. Evaluation strategies range from simple awareness of functional changes to extensive field-based measures (ACSM). Lifestyle activities include examples of activities that can substitute for walking, cycling, and swimming. Elastic refers to elastic cords or bands, free weights include anything that can be held or attached to the wrist or ankles. Body weight includes use of body weight for resistance, stair climbing, chair stands, and push-ups. Physical activity programs and behaviour counselling in older adults populations .Medicine and Science in sports and exercise 2004 M Ealine Cress, David M. Buchner, Thomas Prohaska, James Rimmel, Marybeth Brown, Carol Macera, Loretta DePietro, Wojtek Chodzko-Zajko.

According to the latest recommendations resistance training exercises should not be shorter than 10 minutes, while 2-3 series of exercises of 10-12 repetitions each can enhance muscular strength; exercises aiming to improve flexibility should be undertaken at least 2 times *per* week.

In order to improve the compliance to physical activity programs among the elderly it is fundamental to involve family members and friends. Furthermore, the subject should play an active role in choosing the type of exercise. It is also important to tailor type and intensity of exercise to the condition of the single subject, in order to avoid unrealistic goals. The use of positive reinforce techniques could further improve adherence. In the long run, the risk of accidents and injuries related to physical activity is much lower than the expected benefits (Physical activity programs and behaviour counselling in older adults populations .Medicine and Science in sports and exercise 2004 M Ealine Cress, David M. Buchner, Thomas Prohaska, James Rimmel, Marybeth Brown, Carol Macera, Loretta DePietro, Wojtek Chodzko-Zajko), thus there are no contraindications, a part from those previously listed, to physical activity programs, even among the elderly.

The benefits of exercise in subjects with chronic pathologies extend to include a reduction in mortality and morbidity, an improvement of performance and in the activities of daily living, resulting in greater autonomy and better quality of life. In the elderly, it is easier to promote physical activity by identifying programs and exercises that suit age and functional capacities of these subjects. However, this approach has been often overlooked by health-care workers and the potential benefits of tailored physical activity programs are rarely taken into account by health policies. It could be useful to provide our health-care systems with classifications and algorithms that, by evaluating the functional reserve of the patient, can help defining which program fits best his condition (A little exercise, Journal of Gerontology 2006 vol 61° no 11, 1154-1156. Luigi Ferrucci and Eleanor M.Simonsick).

REFERENCES

A 3-years longitudinal study on body composition changes in the elderly; role of physical exercise. *Clin. Nurt.* 2006Aug; 25: 573-80. Raguso CA, Kyle U, Kossovsky MP, Roynette C, Paoloni-Giacobino A, Hans D, Genton L, Pichard C

A little exercise, *Journal of Gerontology* 2006 vol 61° no 11, 1154-1156. Luigi Ferrucci and Eleanor M.Simonsick

A Prospective Study of walking is compared with vigorous exercise in the prevention of coronary heart disease in women; *The New England Journal of Medicine,* 26 august 1999, Manson E., Frank B., Janet W., Rich-Edwards, Graham A.Colditz, Meir J. Stampfer,Walter C.Willet, Frank E. Speizer, Charles H.Hennekens

A Randomized trial comparino aerobic exercise and resistance exercise with a healt education program in older adults with knee osteoarthritis and seniors trial. *JAMA.* 1997;277:25-31. Ettinger WH, Burns R, Messier SP et al

Adiposity as Compared with Physical Activity in Predicting Mortality among Women, Frank B. Hu, M.D., Walter C. Willett, M.D., Tricia Li, M.D., Meir J. Stampfer, M.D.,Graham A. Colditz, M.D. and JoAnn E. Manson, M.D. *New England Journal of Medicine.* 351, 23 december 2004

American Geriatrics Society Panel on Exercise and Osteoarthritis pain: consensus practice raccomandations. Supplement to the AGS Clinical Practice Guidelines on the management of cronic pain in older adults; *J. Am. Geriatr. Soc.* 2001;49:808-23

Associations of physical activity with body weight and fat in men and women. *Int. J. Obes.* 2001;25:914-919. Ball K, Owen N, Salmon J, Barman A,Gore CJ

Benefits of exercise for community dwelling older adults; *Arch. Phys. Med. Rehabil. Vol.* 85, Suppl 3, July 2004.Jonathan f. bean, MD, MS,Ariona Vora, MD, Walter R.Frontera, MD

Body mass, Fitness and Survival in Veteran Patients: Another Obesità Paradox? *The American Journal of Medicine.* 2007, 120,518-524, Paul McAuley, Jonathan Myers, Joshua Abella, Victor Froelicher

Changes in Leisure-time Physical Activity and Risk of Death: an observational study of 7000 mMen and Women, *American Journal of Epidemiology.* 2003, 158,639, Peter Schnohr, Henrik Scharling, and Jan Skov Jensen

Change in Motor Function and Risk of Mortality in Older Persons; American Geriatrics Society, G*en.* 2007, 55:11-19,Aron S. Buchman, Robert S. Wilson, Patricia A.Boyle, Julia L. Bienias, David A.Bennet

Diabetes and physical disability among older US adults. *Diabetes Care.* 2000; 23:1272-7. Gregg EW, Beckls GL, Williamson DF, Leveille SG, Langlois JA, Engelgau MM et al

Does Late-Life Physical Activity or Exercise Prevent or Minimize Disablement? *Am. J. Prev. Med.* 2003;25:129-136. Julie J. Keysor PhD,PT

Does walking decrease the risk of cardiovascular disease hospitalizations and death in older adults? *J. Am. Geriatr. Soc.* 1996;44:113-20. La Croix AZ, Leveille SG, Hecht JA, Grothaus LC, Wagner EH

Effect of exercise on glycemic control and body mass in type 2 diabetes mellitus: a meta-analysis of controlled clinical trias; *JAMA.* 2001 286:1218-27.Boule NG, Haddad E, Kenny GP, Wells GA, Sigal RJ

Effect of exercise on total intra-abdominal body fat in postmenopausal women: a randomized rail. *JAMA.* 2003, 289:323-330. Irwin ML, Yasui Y, Ulrich CM, Bowen D, Rudolph RE, Schwartz RS, Yukawa M, Aiello E, Potter JD, McTiernam A

Effect of strength and power training on physical function in community-dwelling older adults. *J. Gerontol. A Biol. Sci. Med. Sci.* 2003;58:171-5. Miszko TA, Cress ME; Slade JM, Covei CJ, Agraval SK Doerr CE

Effectiveness of exercise therapy in patients with osteoarthritis of the tip or knee: a systematic review of randomized clinical trials. *Arthritis Rheum.* 1999;42: 1361-9. Van Baar ME, Assendelft WJ, Dekker J, Oostendorp RA, Bijlsma JW

Effects of Walking on Mortality Among non smoking retired men Ami A Hakim MS, Elen Petrovitch MD, Cecil M Burchfiel PhD, G. Webster Ross MD, Beatriz L. Rodriguez MD PhD, Lon R White MD, Katsuhico Yano MD, David Curb MD, and Robert D Abbott MD. *New England Journal of Medicine.* 338, 94-99, 8 january 1998

Exercise comes of age: rationale and reccomandation for a geriatric exercise prescription. *J. Gerontol. Med. Sci.* 2002; 57:262-82. Fiatarone Singh MA

Exercise Standard .A statement for healthcare professionals from the American Heart Association. Writing Group. *Circulation.* 1995;91:580-615.Fletcher GF, Balady G, Froelicher VF, Hartley LH, Haskell WL, Pollock ML

Exercise training as a therapy for chronic heart failure:can older people benefit? *J. Am. Geriatr. Soc.* 2003;51:699-709. Witham MD, Struthers AD, McMurdo ME

Exercise training improves overall physical fitness and quality of life in older women with coronary artery disease, *CHEST.* 2004; 126:1026-1031; Chihya Hung, Bill Daub, Bill Black, Robert Welsh, Arthur Quinney and Mark Haykowsky

Exercise-based rehabilitation for coronary heart disease. *Cochrane Database Syst. Rev.* 2001;CD 001800.Jolliffe JA,Rees K, Taylor RS, Thompson D,Oldridge N, Ebrahim S

Expalining the sex difference in coronary heart disease mortalità among patients with tipe 2 diabetes mellitus: a meta-analysis. *Arch. Intern. Med.* 2002; 162: 1737-45. Kanaya AM, Grady D, Barret-Connor E

Falls prevention over 2 years: a randomized controlled trial in women 80 years and older. *Age Ageing.* 1999;28: 513-8. Compobell AJ, Robertson MC, Gordner MM, Norton RN, Buchner DM

Home-based exercise improves functional performance and quality of lie in women with diastolic heart failure; *Heart Lung.* 2004 Jul-Aug;33:210-8. Gary RA, Sueta CA, Dougherty M, Rosemberg B, Cheek D, Preisser J, Neelon V, McMurray R

Impact of cardiovascular fitness and physical activity level on health outcomes in older persons, *Mechanisms of ageing and developement,* 2003, 259-267. Isabelle J. Dionne, Philip A Ades, Eric T Poehlman

Invecchiare in salute, I risultati di una Ricerca-Intervento sull'efficacia dei corsi di ginnastica per anziani a Torino, Regione Piemonte, 2004

Modifiable Lifestyle Factors and the Metabolic Syndrom in Older Men: Effects of Lifestyle Changes, *Journal of the American Geriatrics Society,* vol 54 issue 12, december 2006, 1909-1914S Goya Wannamethee, A Gerald Shaker, Peter H Whincup

Physical activity among adults > or= 50 yr with or without disabilities; BRFSS 2001; *Med. Sci. Sports Exerc.*2005;37:620-629.Brown DR,Yore MM, Ham SA, Macera CA

Physical activity and cognition in old age; *Current Opinion in Psychiatry.* 2006;19:190-193; Nicola T. Lavtenschloger and Osvaldo P.Almeida

Physical activity and its impact on health outcomes. Prevention of unhealthy weight gain and obesità by physical activity: an analysis of the evidence. *Obesity reviews.* 3 2002, 273-287. J.Erlichman, A. L.Kerbey and WPT James

Physical activity and the prevention of cardiovascular disease. *Curr. Atheroscler. Rep.* 5 2003;299-299-307. Bassuk SS, Manson JE

Physical activity programs and behaviour counselling in older adults populations. *Medicine and Science in sports and exercise.* 2004 M Ealine Cress, David M. Buchner, Thomas Prohaska, James Rimmel, Marybeth Brown, Carol Macera, Loretta DePietro, Wojtek Chodzko-Zajko

Physical activity, functional limitations, and disability in older adults. *J. Am. Geriatr. Soc.* 2000;48:1264-72. Miller ME, Rejeski WJ, Reboussin BA, Ten Have TR, Ettinger WH

Physical activity, including walking, and cognitive function in older women. *JAMA.* 2004 sep 22;292:1454-61. Weuve J, Kang JH, Manson JE, Breteler MM, Ware JH, Grodstein F.

Physiological outcomes of aerobic exercise training in hemiparetic stroke patients. *Stroke.* 1995;26:101-5.Potempa K, Lopez M, Braun LT, Szidon JP,Fogg L, Tincknell T

Physycal Activity by presence and type of functional deficits in older women: the Women's Healt and Aging Studies; *J. of Gerontology.* 2006, vol 61, no 11, 1171-1176, Gerald J.Jerome, Thomas A.Glass, Micelle Miele, Qian-Li Xue, Ross E.Andersen, Linda P.Field)

Power of outcomes measurements to detect clinically significant changes in pulmonary rehabilitation of patients with COPD. *Chest.* 2002; 121:1092-8.De Torres JP, Pinto-Plota V, Ingenito E et al.

Primary Prevention of Coronary Heart Disease in women througth diet and lifestyle Meir J Stampfer M.D., Frank B HU M.D., Joanne Manson M.D., Eric B Rimm, SC.D., and Walter C Willet M.D., *New England Juornal of Medicine.* 2000, 343:16-22

Progressive Resistence exercise and resting blood pressure:a meta-analysis of randomized controlled trials. *Hypertension.* 2000;35:838-43. Kelley GA,Kelley KS

Progressive resistence stength training for physical disability in older people, The Cochrane Library, 2003. Latham N, Anderson CS, Bennett D, Stretton C

Relationship of walking to mortalità among US adults with diabetes. *Arch. Int. Med.* 2003;163:1440-7. Gregg EW, Gerzoff RB, Caspersen CJ, Williamson DF, Narayan KM

The effects of exercise training on elderly persons with cognitive impairment and dementia; a meta-analysis; *Arch. Phys. Med. Rehabil.* 2004;85:1694-1704.Heyn P, Abrev BC, Ottenbacher Kj

Walking decreased risk of cardiovascular disease mortality in older adults with diabetes. *Journal of Clinical Epidemiology.* 60 2007 309-317. Tyler C. Smith, Deborah L. Wingard, Besa Smith, Donna Kritz-Silvestein, Elizabeth Barrett-Connor

In: Exercise and Women's Health
Editor: Laura A. Charlington, pp. 67-97
ISBN: 978-1-60456-013-8

Chapter 3

EFFECTIVENESS OF A WORKPLACE PHYSICAL EXERCISE INTERVENTION ON THE FUNCTIONING, WORK ABILITY, AND SUBJECTIVE WELL-BEING OF WOMEN OFFICE WORKERS – A CLUSTER RANDOMISED CONTROLLED CROSS-OVER TRIAL

T. Sjögren[1], K. Nissinen[2], M. Ojanen[3], H. Vanharanta[4], A. Heinonen[1] and E. Mälkiä[1]

[1] Department of Health Sciences, University of Jyväskylä, Finland
[2] Department of Mathematics and Statistics, University of Jyväskylä, Finland
[3] Department of Psychology, University of Tampere, Finland
[4] Leeds Musculoskeletal Service, Leeds England

ABSTRACT

Background and objectives: Physical exercise interventions are commonly used in the workplace to promote employees' physical and psychosocial functioning and work ability. However, there is limited scientific evidence of the effectiveness of such programmes, especially by gender. Also facts of dose-response effects on functioning or work ability are not yet fully understood. The aim of this study was to investigate among women office workers the effects of workplace physical exercise intervention on physical and psychosocial functioning, work ability, and general subjective well-being. Study is subgroup analyze of larger workplace intervention study.

Methods: 66 volunteer women [mean age 45.4 (SD 8.6) years] employees from four municipal administrative departments of Finland took part in a 15 weeks' cluster randomised cross-over design intervention. The intervention period consisted of light resistance training [30% 1RM (repetition maximum)] with guidance. The no-intervention period did not include any training or guidance. During the first five-week training period the training frequency was once in each working day, and thereafter 7-8 times a week. Musculoskeletal symptoms were measured using the Borg CR10 scales and muscular strength with a 5RM test. Psychosocial functioning, work ability and well-being variables were assessed by descriptive visual rating scales (0-100). Physical activity during the intervention was monitored by a weekly diary (training sessions and training time in minutes). Physical activity outside the intervention was recorded by the one-month all-time recall questionnaire (work, commuting, leisure time and miscellaneous time). The type of activity, frequency, duration and intensity of physical activity were converted to metabolic equivalent (MET) values. Statistical analyses were based on linear mixed models (SAS software). Subgroups analyses of women consisted of employees' who had restricted participation in daily activities because of musculoskeletal symptoms.

Results: Average training time was 122 minutes per 5-week (24 minutes/week, 5 minutes/working day). Load of training was average 342.0 MET minutes per 5-week. Compared with the non-intervention period the physical exercise intervention, resistance training and guidance together significantly decreased among subgroups of women employees' the intensity of headache [(p=0.004), mean difference 0.6 CR10, average percentual change 46%] and neck symptoms [(p=0.023), 0.3 CR10, 42%]. Whereas the active component of the intervention, light resistance training, resulted in significantly reduced intensity of symptoms in shoulder [(p=0.050), 0.27 CR10, 11%] and low back [(p=0.028), 0.45 CR10, 27%] symptoms. The light resistant training improved subjective physical well-being [(p=0.016), 5 units, 7%], physical condition [(p= 0.003), 6 units, 11%] and working ability [(p=0.045), 3 units, 3%,], but it did not affect the other psychosocial functioning and general well-being variables.

Conclusion: A physical exercise intervention, which included daily light resistance training, conducted during the working day affected on functioning and work ability in a positive direction among women office workers. A better understanding of physical exercise intervention's dose-response effects among women employees' can be helpful in maintaining functioning and work ability and preventing impairment in sedentary occupations.

Keywords: CR10, dose-response, exercise, functioning, ICF, metabolic equivalent, musculoskeletal symptoms, physical activity, occupational health, rehabilitation, sedentary work, well-being, women, work ability.

1. Introduction

In general, women and older subjects had more musculoskeletal diseases and symptoms than men and younger subjects (Ekberg et al. 1995, Seistamo and Klockars 1997, Mäkelä et al. 1991, Eriksen et al. 1998, Bovim et al. 1994, Ilmarinen 1999, Hellsing and Bryngelsson 2000, KTL 2004, Strazdins and Bammer 2004). Subjects who were middle aged or women also had more psychosocial troubles and disabilities (Eriksen 1998, KTL 2004, STM 2004). The prevalence of subjective health complaints, like musculoskeletal symptoms, depressive mood, tiredness, and worry, is high in the northern European countries. Women were three times as likely as men to have multiple complaints (Eriksen 1998).

Among the Finnish population over the past 20 years chronic low back and neck syndromes have become less frequent, but self-reported pain in back and neck and weight-bearing joints are equally frequent in Finns of working age today as they were 20 years ago. For example the prevalence of back pain experienced (>30 years) during the past month among women was 36% and among men 30%. The corresponding values for neck pain were 40% and 26% and for shoulder pain 40% and 23% (STM 2004). Although the prevalence of musculoskeletal symptoms has been found to be higher in physically demanding occupations than in physically light occupations (Tola et al. 1988, Luoma et al. 2000, TTL 2000 and

2003), the prevalence of symptoms in the latter occupation has also been rather high, especially in the neck, shoulders, upper extremities and low back area (Linton and Kamwendo 1989, Tola et al 1988, Luoma et al. 2000, Thorbjörnsson et al. 2000, Forsman et al. 2002).

According to the Health 2000 study the majority of the Finnish population feels psychologically quite well. Only 5% in the age groups 30 or over reported a major depressive episode during the past 12 months. Major depressive episodes were more common among women (7%) than among men (4%), and the highest prevalence was found in the working age group (KTL 2004). In the year 2000 among the Finnish working population 35% experienced feelings of mental stress at work, which was slightly less than three years before (TTL 2003). However, the Finnish Health 2000 study reported that among those in gainful employment 25% suffered from mild and 2.5% from severe burnout (STM 2004). Women, compared to Finnish men, have reported more experience of feelings of mental stress at work and a worse work atmosphere. In addition women's mental stress is reported to increase with age (Seistamo and Klockars 1997, TTL 2000 and 2003). Public administration employees reported the worst working atmosphere, with 28% reporting that their working atmosphere was strained, while the corresponding mean value for all occupations was 19% (TTL 2003).

Strazdins and Bammer (2004) investigated Public Service employees IN ??? (73% women and 73% clerical workers) and found gender differences in risk factors. Women's working conditions were more likely to involve physically repetitive work demands. For example, 34% of women compared to 21% of men sat in the same position for long periods of time, 81% of women compared to 73% of men worked longer than 5 hours per day on a computer, and 30% of women compared to 16% of men reported that their job involved repetitive movements all of the time. Women were also more likely to work in poorly designed and uncomfortable environments. 15% of women compared to 10% of men described their work environments as either uncomfortable or very uncomfortable. In addition, women spent considerably less time than men exercising or relaxing during leisure-time. 20% of women did not exercise at all and 14% did not spend time relaxing, over the previous month. This compares to 12% and 10%, respectively, for men. Women gender (Bergqvist et al. 1995, Ekberg et al. 1995, Hakkarainen et al. 2001, Viikari-Juntura et al. 2001) and sedentary working positions (Fredriksson et al. 2000, TTL 2003,) was determined to be risk factors for musculoskeletal symptoms also in other studies.

Hales et al. (1994) and Fogelman and Lewis et al. (2002) successes that among VDT workers the main foci in reducing musculoskeletal symptoms are workstation ergonomics, the need to limit the number of uninterrupted hours at the keyboard and the psychosocial work environment. Linton and van Tulder (2001) suggest that workplace programs should assess risk and be tailored to the risk profile of individual or the workplace. Many previous studies have recommended performing more randomised, controlled trials of high methodological quality at work place. Internal validity scores like randomization, treatment allocation, drop-out rate, blinding, intention-to-treat analysis, relevant outcome measures and definition of the intervention should be taken into account (Shephard 1996, Drisman et al. 1998, Proper et al. 2002, Proper et al. 2003, Liddle et al. 2004, van Poppel et al. 2004, Tveito et al. 2004, Dworking et al. 2005).

The main idea behind our physical exercise intervention was to counterbalance office workers sedentary work or to obtain relief from monotonous and fixed working positions and to investigate the effects of a 15-week physical exercise intervention on the intensity of headache and neck, shoulder and low back symptoms, as well as on psychosocial functioning, work ability and subjective general well-being of women office workers. Framework of the study was International Classification of Functioning, Disability and Health (ICF).

2. Material and Methods

2.1. Subjects, Study Designs and Randomization in the CRT Study

At the level of the cluster the criterion for inclusion was physically light work performed by workers in various departments of the City of Kuopio's central administration. Average intensity of occupational physical activity (OPA) was 1.5 metabolic equivalent (MET) measured according to MetPro® questionnaires (Sjögren 2006). Four different-sized departments, with a combined population of 123 office workers were selected. 90 volunteer workers (73%) from the four departments took part in the physical exercise intervention [66 women and, 24 men, mean age 45.7 (SD 8.5) years]. The volunteers' level of education was mainly college or university (86%), and they had spent an average of 13 years in their current workplace. The volunteers` state of health was assessed in collaboration with an occupational health physician, and was based on the answers given to the working ability index questionnaire and the intensity of pain or discomfort experienced during the past 7 days. None of the subjects met the exclusion criteria, which were as follows: difficult or neglected diseases, acute injury, postoperative state, inflammation, or neurological signs (Sjögren-Rönkä et al. 2002).

Among the population of office workers the most common areas of musculoskeletal complaint in the 12-month and 7-day recall were shoulders, head, neck and low back. Women reported more symptoms in the shoulders and low back in the 12-month recall and 7-day recall and the intensity of symptoms were higher among women than men in the shoulders and low back area. The level of psychosocial functioning and work ability of the women and men study populations were quite high, but in the 12-month recall women had worse psychosocial functioning than men; women had more somatic symptoms and anxiety than men and worse physical condition, self-confidence, mood and meaning of life than men. The older workers (46 years≥) did not differ substantially from their younger counterparts. (Sjögren-Rönkä et. al 2001). Table 1 gives physical and psychological functioning, work ability, social environmental factors at work and general subjective well-being means and standard deviations by gender. The ICF terminology was used in separating different domains.

Table 1. Physical and psychological functioning, work ability, social environmental factors at work and general subjective well-being means and standard deviations by gender

	Mean (SD)			
	All (n=90)	Women (n=66)	Men (n=24)	p-value
Age, years	45.7 (8.6)	45.4 (8.6)	46.6 (8.6)	0.559
Height, cm	167.7 (7.7)	164.5 (5.7)	176.3 (5.5)	0.000
Weight, kg	71.3 (13.2)	67.7 (11.4)	81.2 (13.1)	0.000
Current workplace, years	12.7 (8.5)	13.1 (9.4)	12.7 (8.1)	0.856
PHYSICAL FUNCTIONING				
1. Sensory functions and pain Intensity of musculoskeletal symptoms (0= Noting at all, 10=very,very strong)				
Headache	1.6 (2.1)	1.9 (2.1)	1.0 (2.0)	0.069
Neck symptoms	1.1 (1.9)	1.8 (2.0)	1.1 (1.7)	0.180
Shoulder symptoms	2.0 (2.4)	2.4 (2.4)	1.0 (1.8)	0.004
Low back symptoms	1.4 (2.0)	1.8 (2.3)	0.6 (1.5)	0.005
2. Functions of metabolic system				
Body fat percentage (%)	26.9 (7.2)	29.3 (6.2)	20.3 (4.8)	0.000
3. Neuromusculoskeletal and movement-related functions Strength (kg)				
Hand grip strength				
- Right	41.2 (11.8)	36.8 (7.1)	53.6 (12.7)	0.000
- Left	36.6 (10.7)	32.1 (5.4)	49.4 (11.4)	0.000
Lower extremities muscles				
- Knee extension	49.5 (16.0)	47.9 (13.1)	63.5 (17.3)	0.000
- Knee flexion	58.8 (14.4)	52.3 (9.7)	74.9 (10.6)	0.000
4. Functions of the cardiovascular and respiratory systems Maximum oxygen uptake				
- mL 0_2 x kg^{-1} x min^{-1}	29.1 (8.3)	25.8 (6.3)	38.1 (6.1)	0.000
- MET	8.3 (2.2)		7.2 (1.4)	
Subjective physical condition	62.5 (17.1)	58.8 (15.0)	72.3 (18.9)	0.002
5. Mobility				
Physical activity (MET)				
Leisure time (LTPA)				
- Time-weighted intensity average	3.7 (2.5)	3.6 (1.9)	5.6 (3.1)	0.005
- Maximum intensity	5.1 (3.3)	4.3 (2.4)	6.9 (4.2)	0.019
All activities time (AT)				
- Time-weighted intensity average				
2.0 (0.5)	1.9 (0.6)	2.1 (0.6)	0.388	2.0 (0.5)
- Maximum intensity	6.0 (2.7)	5.3 (1.8)	7.2 (3.9)	0.063
PSYCHOLOGICAL FUNCTIONING AND GENERAL SUBJECTIVE WELL-BEING (0=worst possible, 100= best possible)				
1. Orientation functions				
Self-confidence	72.7 (14.4)	69.0 (14.2)	82.3 (9.6)	0.000
2. Emotional functions				
Anxiety	74.3 (14.2)	71.8 (13.6)	81.1 (13.7)	0.005
3. Carrying out daily routine				
Physical well-bein	77.3 (14.1)	75.7 (14.0)	81.8 (13.8)	0.072
Somatic symptoms	80.1 (14.9)	77.9 (15.6)	86.3 (11.1)	0.018

Table 1. (Continued).

	Mean (SD)			
	All (n=90)	Women (n=66)	Men (n=24)	p-value
Mood	73.3 (15.5)	70.9 (16.3)	79.8 (10.7)	0.015
4. Life satisfaction	74.0 (14.6)	72.4 (14.7)	78.2 (13.6)	0.098
5. Meaning of life	80.7 (15.7)	78.2 (17.1)	87.3 (8.5)	0.009
WORK ABILITY AND SOCIAL ENVIRONMENTAL FACTORS AT WORK (0=worst possible, 100= best possible)				
Work ability	87.4 (9.9)	86.8 (10.3)	90.6 (8.6)	0.115
Mental stress at work	58.2 (22.6)	57.2 (23.3)	61.0 (20.9)	0.483
Working atmosphere	67.5 (21.2)	65.5 (22.5)	73.1 (16.3)	0.134

The physical exercise intervention study was a cluster randomised –controlled cross-over design. We used cluster randomization in our clinical trial for logistic, ethical and financial reasons. We also wanted to minimize contamination between control and treatment groups. In the individual-based randomization the possibility of contamination of control group subjects by extensive daily contact in the workplace with treatment group subjects should be considered.

Baseline measurements were performed before the first intervention period in September, 1999. After the baseline measurements, the "blind" measurers allocated the workers into the two treatment sequence groups, Treatment Group 1 and Treatment Group 2, using cluster randomization. Treatment Group 1 contained clusters 3 and 4, and Treatment Group 2 contained clusters 1 and 2. In the first period (autumn), Treatment Group 1 took part in the intervention while Treatment Group 2 did not. In the second period (spring), the roles were reversed so that now Treatment Group 2 took part in the intervention while Treatment Group 1 did not. The cross-over design was conducted without any washout time between the two treatments periods. Therefore, the second period commenced immediately after the first period in January. Both periods lasted for 15 weeks. The sequence was not revealed until the interventions were assigned.

In this study effectiveness of a workplace physical exercise intervention on the functioning, work ability, and subjective well-being were analysed in a group of women volunteers` [n=66, mean age 45.4 (SD 8.6) years]. In studying the effects of a workplace physical exercise intervention on the intensity of headache and neck, shoulder and low back symptoms in women office workers the criteria for inclusion were headache or pain or discomfort (=symptoms) in the neck, shoulders or low back, which to some degree had restricted participation in daily activities during the 12-month period preceding the intervention. These women were categorized into three partially overlapping sub-groups: the Headache Symptoms Group (n= 33), the Neck Symptoms Group (n=30), the Shoulder Symptoms Group (n=34) and the Low Back Symptoms Group (n=29). The criteria for exclusion from these sub-groups were no restriction in daily activities during the last 12 months due to headache, neck, shoulder or low back symptoms.

Study subjects, cluster randomisation, the cross-over study design and the groups analysed in the study population are presented in a flow chart in figure 1. The flow chart was designed according to Consort statement: extension to cluster randomized trials information by Campbell et al. (2004).

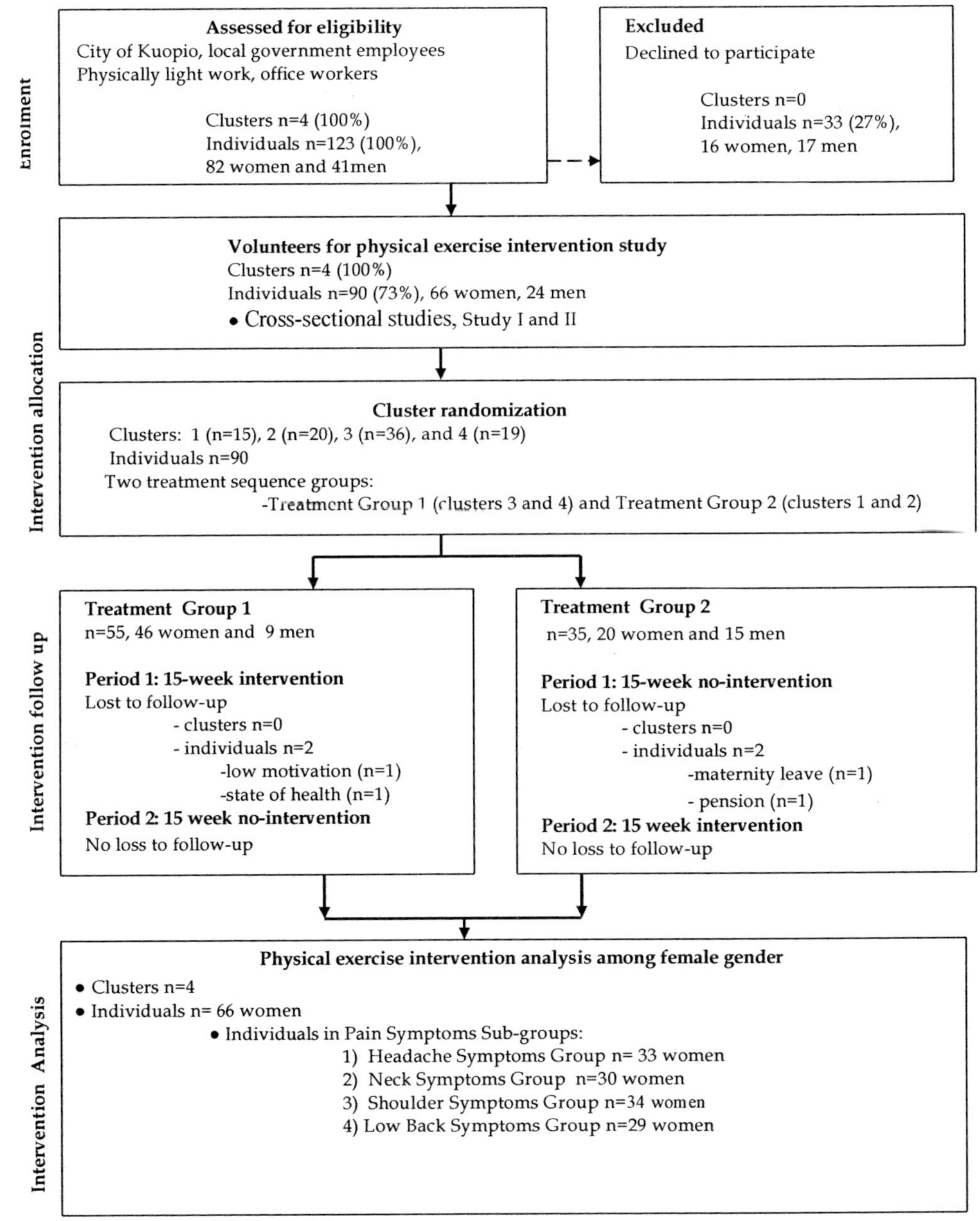

Figure 1. Study design, randomisation, and study subjects in the CRT and follow-up study.

2.2. Measurements

The ICF classification was performed according to the World Health Organization ICF general coding rules. As the functioning of a person can be affected at the body, individual and societal level, the user should always take into consideration components of the classification, namely Body Functions and Structures, Activities and Participation, and Environmental factors. Body Functions are the physiological functions of body systems, including psychological functions. An activity is the execution of a task or action by an individual. Users will select the most salient codes for their purpose to describe a given health experience. Information that reflects the person's feeling of involvement or satisfaction with level of function is currently not coded in (WHO 2001).

2.2.1. Measurements of Body Functions and Structures

Sensory Functions and Pain

Intensity of Musculoskeletal Symptoms

The intensity of musculoskeletal ache, pain, discomfort (= musculoskeletal symptoms) experienced during the previous seven days was measured using the Borg CR10 scale. The scale describes the subjective level of symptoms. The scale varies from "nothing at all" (0) to "extremely strong" (10) symptoms. "Extremely weak" corresponds to 0.5 on the scale and is the threshold of what it is possible to perceive. Subjects start with a verbal expression and then choose a number. The reliability and validity of the Borg CR10 scale are good (Borg, 1998), and it has been recommended for use in exercise studies (ACMS, 2000).

Neuromusculoskeletal and Movement-Related Functions

Strength of Upper and Lower Extremities

The one-repetition maximum (1RM) for the upper and lower extremities was estimated with the sub-maximal 5RM test (McDonagh and Daves, 1984, Braith et al. 1993, ACSM 2000) using air resistance equipment (HUR Ltd, Finland). The standardized test movements were upper extremity extension and flexion and knee flexion and extension. A metronome was used to define the speed of muscular contraction. The average movement performance time for a single repetition of a testing movement was 3.0 seconds. The subjects performed five sets of repetitions with loads of 10 kg, 20 kg, 30 kg etc., until they were unable to perform the defined sets properly. The resting period between the 5RM test sets was 1 minute and between the different test movement stations 3 minutes. The upper extremity extension and flexion and knee flexion and extension 1RM values were estimated according to the 5 RM value according to scheme [(-4.18 x R.M. value of load as percent) + 103] published by McDonagh and Daves (1984). The corresponding 1RM and 30% 1RM was read from the table x.

Self-Confidence and Anxiety

Self-assessed subjective anxiety and self-confidence were measured by descriptive visual rating scales. On the scale, 0 represented the worst possible and 100 the best possible physical well-being, self-confidence or anxiety. 50 represented the neutral position (Ojanen 1994, Ojanen, 2000). In descriptive visual rating scale subjects draw a short line across the vertical line at the point that best corresponds to their self assessment.

2.2.2. Measurements of Activity

Mobility

Physical Activity at Work, and During Commuting, Leisure Time and Miscellaneous Time

Physical activity was measured by the one-month all-time recall questionnaire, where activity was divided into work, commuting, leisure time and miscellaneous time such as gardening or homework. The type of activity, frequency, duration and intensity of physical activity were converted to MET values with the aid of a special computer programme (MetPro®, SciReha Ltd, Jyväskylä, Finland). The intensity of physical activity was assessed on the basis of getting out of breath and sweating (Mälkiä et al. 1994, Mälkiä 1996). One MET represents the approximate rate of 0_2 consumption of a seated individual at rest = 3.5 $mlxkg^{-1}xmin^{-1}$ (ACSM 2000, Howley 2001). In our study we used gross cost of physical activity values, which included the resting metabolic rate and the cost of the activity in OPA, LTPA and all activities time (AT), which included OPA, commuting and LTPA. We used three MET-parameters in our study. First, the time-weighted intensity average (TWA), which was calculated for the activity categories by dividing the sum of MET minutes by the total time in minutes. Second, maximum MET intensity (MMET), which is the highest observed value in the activity categories, and, third, maximal oxygen consumption were expressed as MET values (Mälkiä et al. 1994, Mälkiä 1996, ISO/FDIS 8996, 2004).

Physical Activity During the Physical Exercise Intervention

Physical activity during the physical exercise intervention was measured by a diary. Each subject maintained a weekly diary to record training sessions, including the time in minutes spent performing light resistance training during each session.

General Tasks and Demands

Musculoskeletal Disability

Self-reported restriction on participation in daily activities because of musculoskeletal symptoms experienced during the last 12 months was measured with a modified version of the standardized Nordic questionnaire (Kuorinka 1987). We changed the scale from a dichotomous (yes/no) answers to an ordinal scale (0-4). On the scale, 0 represented situations where there had been no restrictions on daily activities due to certain musculoskeletal symptoms and 4 a situation where there had been a continuous restriction on daily activities due to certain musculoskeletal symptoms during the last 12 months (Andersson et al. 1987).

Somatic Symptoms, Mood, Physical Well-Being and Subjective Physical Condition

Self-estimated subjective somatic symptoms and mood, physical well-being and subjective physical condition were measured by descriptive visual rating scales. On the scale, 0 represented the worst possible and 100 the best possible situation, and 50 represented the neutral position (Ojanen 1994, Ojanen 2000). Somatic symptoms, mood and physical well-being were assessed in relation to work and/or leisure.

2.2.3. Measurements of Participation and Social Work-Related Environmental Factors

Subjective Work Ability

Subjective work ability was measured by descriptive visual rating scales. On the scale, 0 represented the worst possible and 100 the best possible situation, and 50 represented the neutral position (Ojanen 1994, Ojanen 2000).

Mental Stress at Work and Working Atmosphere

Self-estimated subjective mental stress at work and the working atmosphere were measured by descriptive visual rating scales and assessed in relation to the social environment at work. On the scale, 0 represented the worst possible and 100 the best possible situation, and 50 represented the neutral position (Ojanen 1994, Ojanen 2000).

2.2.4. Measurements of General Subjective Well-Being

Subjective Life Satisfaction and Meaning of Life

Self-estimated life satisfaction and meaning of life were measured by descriptive visual rating scales. On the scale, 0 represented the worst possible and 100 the best possible situation, and 50 represented the neutral position (Ojanen 1994, Ojanen 2000). Information that reflects the person's feeling of involvement or satisfaction with level of function is currently not coded in (WHO 2001).

2.2.5. Measurements of Feasibility of the Physical Exercise Intervention

Measurements of feasibility of the physical exercise intervention were measured according measures of adherence. The first of these training sessions adherence is the percentage ratio of self-reported training sessions and guided training sessions. The second, training adherence is the average percentage ratio of self-reported training time and guided target time. Self-reported resistance training time was calculated according to the weekly training diary and target training time was calculated according to the guided training frequency and the average time spent being physically active in a single session (6 minutes).

2.3. Physical Exercise Intervention in CRT Study

The intervention consisted of progressive light resistance training and guidance. The participants were entitled to take time out during the working day to train by themselves in the departments' own training facilities when they felt the need to counterbalance their sedentary work or to obtain relief from monotonous and fixed working positions. The time at which training could be performed during the working day was not restricted. During the first five-week period, the non-supervised light resistance training was to be performed once each working day (5 times a week). During the second and third 5-week periods, the resistance training was to be performed 1-2 times each working day (a total of about 7-8 times a week). Individual training resistances were controlled twice during the 15-week period at the research institute or in the departments' own training facilities. At the department level, a physiotherapist gave three group sessions on how to train and general guidance on postural and movement control.

The resistance training was defined as light according to previous studies (ACSM 1998, Borg 1998, Kaikkonen et al. 2000) and our two pilot studies before the start of the physical exercise intervention. We utilized participants′ perceptions of exertion (Borg RPE 6-20) during light resistance training to set the training load to 30 % of 1RM (repetition maximum) and participants′ opinions to select suitable training equipment for the workplace.

2.3.1. Light Resistance Training

The light resistance training consisted of six dynamic symmetrical movements: upper extremity extension, upper extremity flexion, trunk rotation to the right, trunk rotation to the left, knee extension and knee flexion (figure 2). The training movements were carried out 20 times with a 30-second pause between the training movements. There was no defined sequence between the training movements, except that the physiotherapist recommended that the upper extremity movements' flexion should be performed after extension. The training resistances of 30% of one repetition maximum (1RM) (McDonagh and Daves, 1984) for each movement were estimated at five-week intervals for each individual with a sub-maximal 5RM test performed using air resistance equipment (HUR Ltd, Finland). The training load for the right and left trunk rotation movements was determined from the result for the upper extremity flexion movement. The training load averages during the physical exercise intervention period in upper extremity extension were 10 kilogram (kg) among women, and in upper extremity flexion and trunk rotation to the right and left 14 kg among women. Among women knee extension was 13 kg and knee flexion was 15 kg. The average movement performance time for a single repetition of a training movement was 1.8 seconds and average training time in one light resistance training session was 6.2 minutes. The estimated target training time in minutes per the first 5-week period was 150 minutes and in the second and third periods 210 minutes, the equivalent of 30/42 minutes per week and 6/8 minutes per working day (Sjögren 2006).

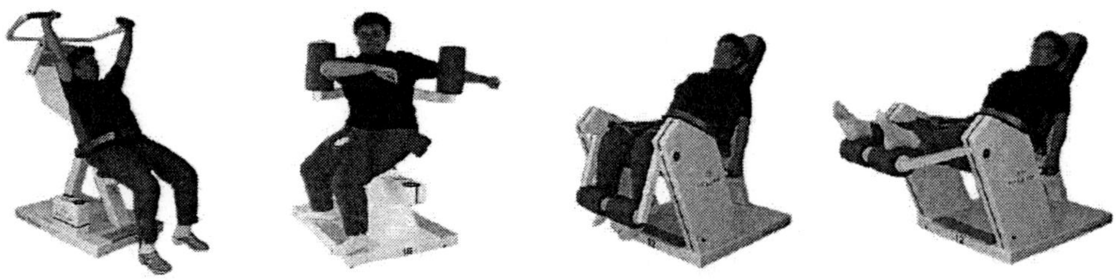

Figure 2. Light resistance training consisted of six dynamic symmetrical movements: upper extremity extension, upper extremity flexion, trunk rotation to the right, trunk rotation to the left, knee extension and knee flexion.

Because we also wanted to ensure that our 30% 1RM resistance training was intensive enough, we conducted a third pilot study at the beginning of the training sessions to measure cardiovascular response (HR, VO_2,RPE) during a light (30% 1RM) exercise session among a similar sedentary occupation population (n=11) (Rönkä 2000). MET values were analyzed using as basic values the 0_2 consumption of a seated individual at rest (3.5 mlxkg^{-1}xmin^{-1}), the heart rate (average 63% HR_{max}) and oxygen consumption (average 35% VO_{2max}), which were measured by the direct method (Cosmed, Italy). The calculated average TWA was 4.2 (SD

1.0) MET during one light resistance training session and the average RPE of all sessions was 12 (SE 0.3). Because in our study population (n=90) the average maximal oxygen uptake in METs was 33% lover than in the pilot study population, the estimated average TWA during one light resistance training session was also lower, being 2.8 (SD 0.7) MET (Sjögren 2006).

2.3.2. Guidance

During the baseline measurement subjects received feedback on their physical functioning from assessors. At the department level, a physiotherapist provided training instructions and general guidance on postural and movement control in three group sessions (3x20 minutes) at 5-week intervals. The subjects learned to use the Borg Rating of Perceived Exertion (RPE 6-20) and pain (CR10) scales (Borg 1998, ACSM 2000) to control their training. The general instruction given was that the perceived exertion should be light (RPE 10-12) and pain levels on the CR10 scale should not temporarily increase by more than one unit from the starting level during an active training session. Moreover, neck, upper extremities and low back position, dynamic muscle contraction, sufficient ranges of motion and respiration were emphasized. Subjects were guided to train under both eyes-open and eyes-closed conditions (Sjögren 2006). Motor control of training movements move from extrinsic feedback (knowledge of performance, knowledge of results) to subjects own intrinsic feedback (muscle force, length, joint position, body position, and vision) (Schmidt 1991). The physiotherapist encouraged the subjects to use the same ergonomic principles: no-loaded positions of neck, upper extremity and low back and dynamic muscle contraction, in work and leisure (Sjögren 2006).

2.3.3. No-Physical Exercise Intervention

During the 15-week no-physical exercise intervention (= no-intervention) period, no light resistance training was performed nor was any guidance provided. The participants simply took part in the measurements.

2.3.4. Avoiding Physical and Psychosocial Co-Interventions

Excluding the light resistance training, the participants were asked to keep the intensity and amount of their physical activity unchanged during the intervention and no-intervention periods. Also, no occupational health services were provided or the subjects were not initiated into new activities in occupational health and safety during the study. Other physical activities were controlled using metabolic equivalent (MET) values. During the interventions, no statistically significant changes in physical activity were found in the time-weighted intensity average or maximum intensity of activity in OPA, LTPA, or in AT in Treatment Groups 1 and 2. As the level of other physical activity performed was not statistically significant, this was not added into the statistical model as a covariate (Sjögren 2006).

2.4. Statistical Analyses in the CRT Study

We used cluster-specific methods because departments rather than individuals were randomized. The effects of the intervention on the physical and psychosocial functioning were analyzed using linear mixed models (Brown and Prescott 1999, Goldstein 1995). This approach has several advantages over traditional analyses such as ANOVA. Firstly, the clustering effect of department can easily be taken into account in the analysis (people within a certain department tend to be homogeneous). Secondly, there is no need to exclude any subject for whom complete data are not obtained, because data lost during the CRT follow-up can be considered random. Thirdly, it is possible to lighten the familiar assumption of equal error variances with mixed models. Randomisation of departments makes the study design hierarchical, as the subjects are nested within departments and treatment groups. It also brings department as a random part of the model.

The main advantage in cross-over designs is that the intervention and no-intervention are compared within subjects, that is, the response of a subject to an intervention will be contrasted with the same subject's response to no-intervention. Removing subject variation in this way makes cross-over trials potentially more efficient than similar-sized, parallel group trials in which each subject is exposed to only one treatment. In principle, exercise effects can be estimated with greater precision given the same number of subjects (Sibbald and Roberts 1998).

The essential features of the cross-over design were modelled as fixed effects: main effects of treatment (intervention or no-intervention), treatment group [Treatment group 1 (order of treatments ab), Treatment group 2 (order of treatments ba)], treatment period (1=autumn, 2= spring) measurements within the treatment period (1-3), as well as their possible interactions. The random part of the model consisted department effects, the effects of individuals within departments, and their (random) interactions with the fixed factors. The random part is required to account for the clustering effects of departments (on individuals) and individuals (on repeated measurements) in order to obtain standard errors and significance tests that correctly reflect features of the design. Time spent performing light resistance training in the current 5-week period (1-3) in minutes and physical and psychosocial functioning measurements at the baseline were added into the model as covariates.

The model described above was estimated and evaluated first. Then we hierarchically simplified this original model as far as possible by removing the non-significant effects one by one, beginning with the most complex least significant interactions. The model that could not be simplified any further without dropping a significant effect or violating the hierarchy principle (that is, non-significant lower-order effects cannot be removed if a significant higher-order interaction of the same factors is present) was then evaluated against the original model using the Akaike information criterion (AIC) (Sakamoto et al., 1986). If it appeared to fit the data better than the original model, it was selected as the final one. Otherwise we used the original model.

The estimation and significance testing was carried out by the MIXED procedure in the SAS software (SAS 1999), which involved the restricted maximum likelihood (REML) method of estimation (Patterson and Thompson 1971) with related F tests. The estimates from the final model were used in calculating the confidence intervals (CI) and performing the significance tests for the effects of the physical exercise interventions.

The effects of the physical exercise intervention on other physical activity performed outside it were evaluated using the same statistical principles as for physical and psychosocial functioning, using linear mixed models (Brown and Prescott 1999, Goldstein 1995).

2.5. Ethical Concerns

The study was approved by the ethical committee of the University of Kuopio and the University Hospital of Kuopio.

3. Results

3.1. The Feasibility of the CRT Physical Exercise Intervention

Among the women office workers (n=66) measures of adherence were conducted. The first, according to the weekly questionnaire, the self-reported adherence average during a 5-week period was 17 times, which was 53% of the guided sessions. The second, self-reported training time adherence average during a 5-week period was 122 minutes, which was 64% of the estimated target minutes, according to the 6 minutes average training time in one light resistance training session. The self reported and guided mean training sessions, training times (in minutes and MET minutes) and adherence percentage ratios during the intervention according to the training periods are presented in table 2. The third, according to our note, women participated average two times in the training guidance sessions.

Table 2. Mean numbers of training sessions, mean training times in minutes and MET minutes as well as adherence percentage ratios during the intervention among women office workers

Periods	Self-reported	Guided	Adherence %
First 5-week	15	25	60
Second 5-week	21	35	60
Third 5-week	15	35	43
Total 15-week	51	95	54
Average during 5-week	17	32	53

Average number of training minutes of light resistance training					
	Self-reported		Estimated target ‡		Adherence %
Periods	minutes* / MET min †		minutes / MET min †		
First 5-week	109.9	307.7	150	420	73.3
Second 5-week	143.8	402.6	210	588	68.5
Third 5-week	112.4	342.7	210	588	53.5
Total 15-week	366.2	1025.4	570	1596	64.3
Average during 5- week	122.1	341.9	190	532	64.3

* Light resistance training time in minutes during the intervention (15 weeks) in 5-week periods

† MET minutes were calculated according to TWA 2.8 METs.

‡ Estimated target training time in minutes in 5-week periods: first period, 5 sessions x 6 minutes x 5 weeks = 150 minutes; second and third period, 7 sessions x 6 minutes x 5 weeks = 210 minutes.

The average estimated MET hours (METh) during light resistance training over 5 weeks was 5.8 METh, which was 1.5% of AT (383.2 METh) and 8.7% of LTPA (64.4 METh). The

MET hours during 15 weeks' light resistance training and its percentage proportions of AT and LTPA is presented in the framework of physical activity, in figure 3.

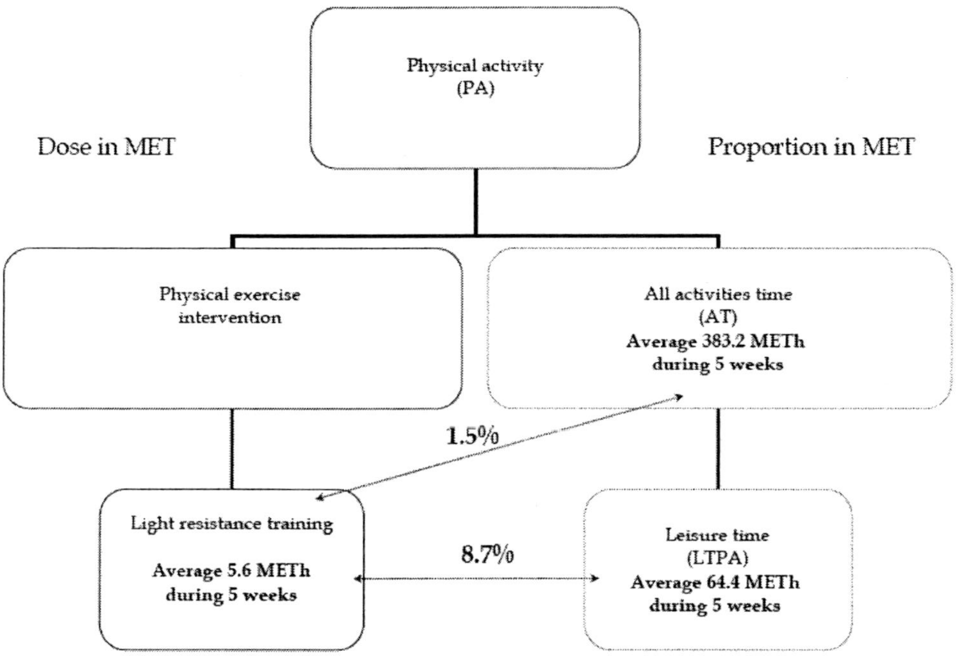

Figure 3. Light resistance training as percentage of LTPA and AT among women office workers.

3.2. Effectiveness of a CRT Workplace Physical Exercise Intervention on the Functioning, Work Ability, and Subjective Well-Being of Office Workers

3.2.1. Effectiveness of a CRT Workplace Physical Exercise Intervention on Body Functions and Structures

Effects of Workplace Physical Exercise Intervention on Intensity of Headache and Neck and Shoulder Symptoms in the Subgroups

Women subgroups were formed at the individual level, the criteria being headache or symptoms in the neck, which to some degree had restricted participation in daily activities during the 12-month period preceding the intervention. In the Headache Symptoms group (n=33) the physical exercise intervention, resistance training and guidance together significantly decreased the intensity of headache (p=0.004), and also in the Neck Symptoms groups (n=30) the intensity of neck symptoms decreased (p=0.023) following the intervention. In the Shoulder Symptoms group (n=34) nearly significant effect (p=0.050) of physical light resistance training on the shoulder area was found.

The estimated mean intensity of headache in the CR10 during the intervention was 0.70 (SE 0.13), and during the no-intervention period 1.27 (SE 0.17), the mean difference being -

0.62 (95% CI -0.20, -1.0). Compared to the corresponding no-intervention period, the intervention led to a 49% (95% CI 16, 82) decrease in the intensity of headache.

The estimated mean intensity of neck symptoms in the CR10 during the intervention was 0.46 (SE 0.11), and during the no-intervention period 0.78 (SE 0.14), the mean difference being -0.33 (95% CI -0.05, -0.61). Compared to the corresponding no-intervention period, the intervention led to a 42% (95% CI 6, 79) decrease in the intensity of neck symptoms. Figures 4 and 5 present the observed mean intensity of symptoms and standard deviations (SD) for headache and neck and symptoms at the baseline, and during the intervention and no-intervention periods.

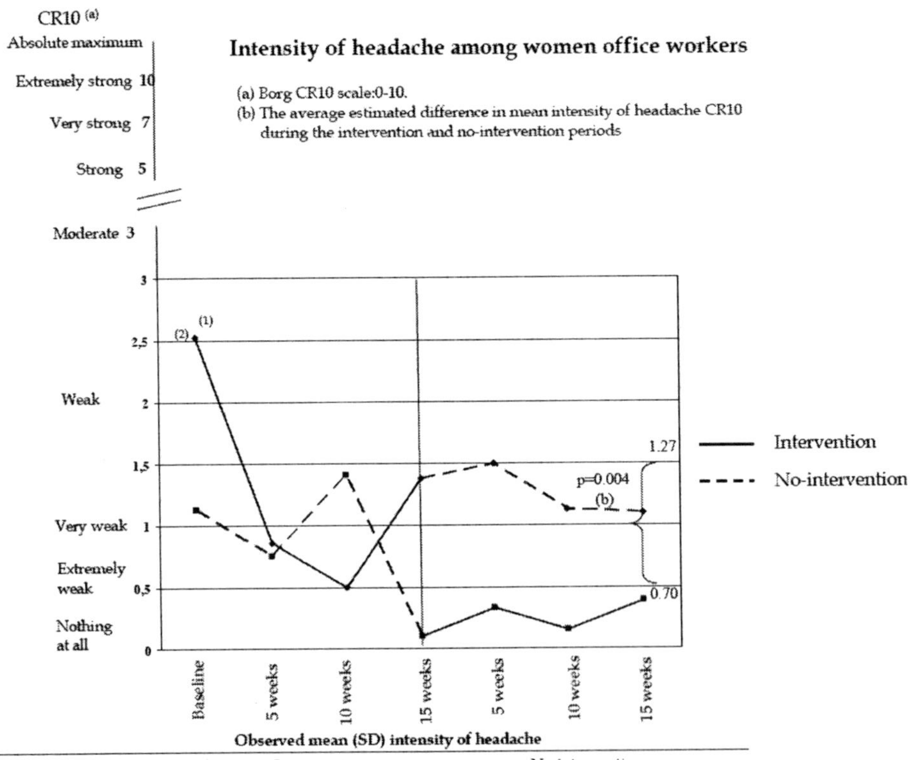

	Baseline	Intervention			No-intervention		
Treatment Group 1 (1) n=23	2.52 (2.36)	0.86 (1.28)	0.50 (1.28)	1.38 (1.75)	1.50 (2.14)	1.13 (1.54)	1.10 (1.70)
	Baseline	No-intervention			**Intervention**		
Treatment Group 2 (2) n=10	1.13 (1.80)	0.75 (1.49)	1.40 (1.58)	0.10 (0.32)	0.33 (1.00)	0.15 (0.34)	0.39 (1.08)

Figure 4. Observed mean intensity of symptoms and standard deviations (SD) for headache at the baseline, and during the intervention and no-intervention periods.

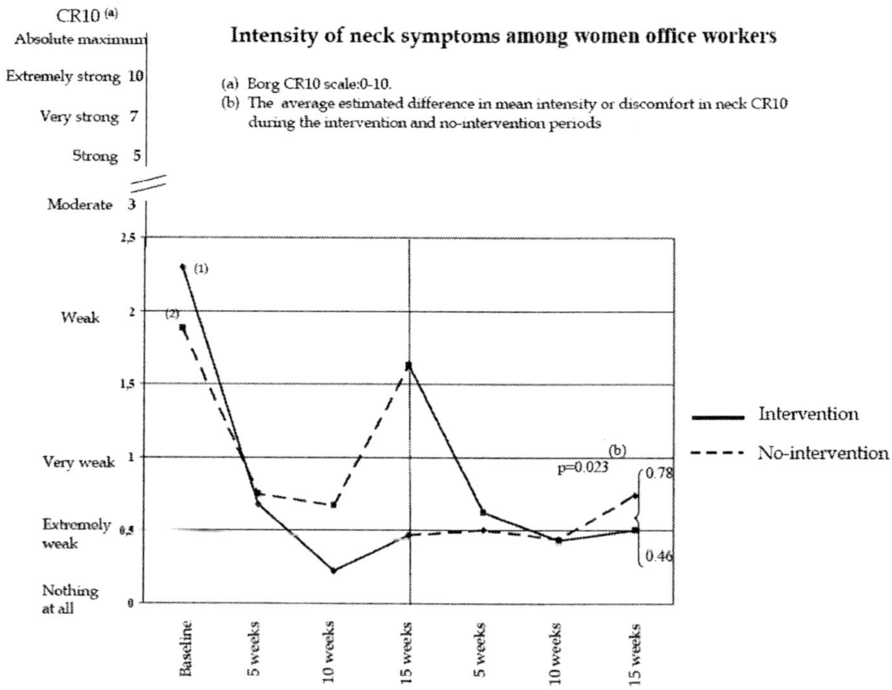

Observed mean (SD) of neck symptoms

	Baseline	Intervention			No-intervention		
Treatment Group 1 (1)	2.30 (2.35)	0.68 (1.20)	0.22 (0.65)	0.47 (1.12)	0.50 (1.10)	0.44 (0.92)	0.74 (1.19)
n=22	Baseline	No-intervention			**Intervention**		
Treatment Group 2 (2)	1.88 (2.05)	0.75 (1.49)	0.67 (1.63)	1.63 (1.92)	0.62(1.19)	0.43 (1.13)	0.50 (0.93)
n=8							

Figure 5. Observed mean intensity of symptoms and standard deviations (SD) for neck symptoms at the baseline, and during the intervention and no-intervention periods.

Effects of Workplace Physical Exercise Intervention on Intensity of Low Back Symptoms in the Subgroups

Subgroups were formed at the individual level, the criteria being low back symptoms which to some degree had restricted participation in daily activities during the 12-month period preceding the intervention (n=29). The active component of the intervention, light resistance training, resulted in significantly ($p=0.028$) reduced intensity of symptoms in the low back (figure 6). The average estimated reduction in low back symptoms was calculated from the regression coefficient: -0.00365 (95% CI -0.00042972, -0.00687028). The regression coefficient indicates the reduction in symptoms if one minute is added to the training time during a given 5-week period. During the 5-week period, the average reduction in low back symptoms was 0.30 CR10 (95% CI 0.05, 0.84) when the average training time during the 5-week period was 122 minutes (24 minutes per week, 5 minutes per working day). The intervention, ignoring the time spent performing light resistance training, did not have a significant effect on the intensity of low back symptoms.

According to the 0.30 CR10 value, in Treatment Group 1 the estimated average reduction was 17% (95% CI 2, 31) compared to the baseline measurement (2.7/CR10). In Treatment Group 2, it was 37% (95% CI 4, 69) compared to the last no-intervention measurement (1.21/CR10). Figure x presents the observed mean and standard deviations (SD) for the intensity of low back symptoms at the baseline and during the intervention and no-intervention periods.

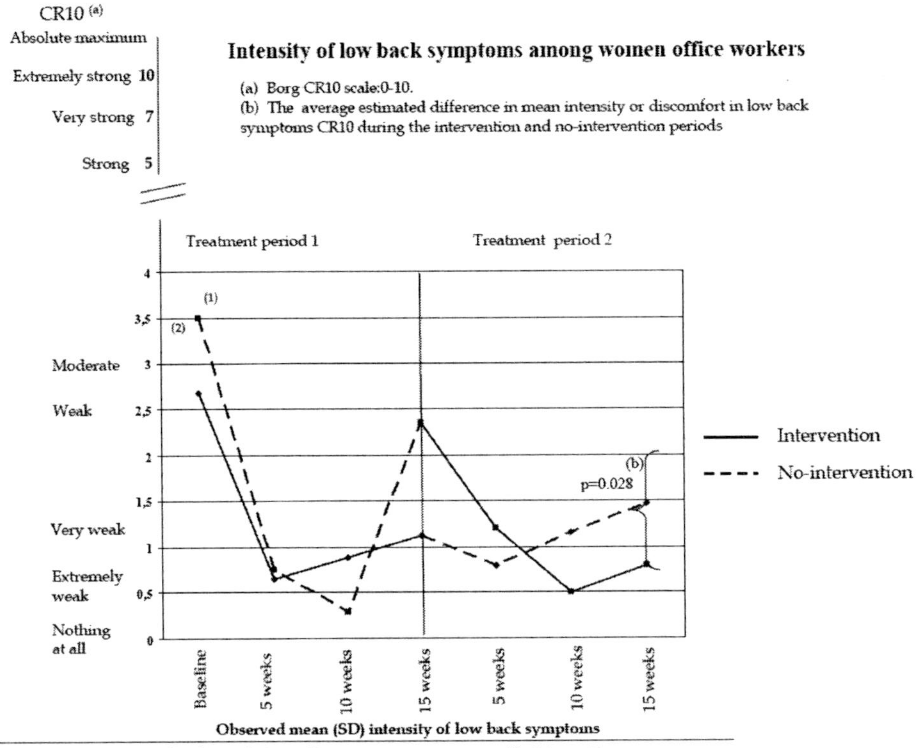

Observed mean (SD) intensity of low back symptoms

	Baseline	Intervention			No-intervention		
Treatment Group 1 (1) n=19	2.68 (1.87)	0.65 (1.41)	0.88 (1.76)	1.12(1.93)	0.79 (1.25)	1.15 (2.10)	1.47 (2.12)
	Baseline	No-intervention			**Intervention**		
Treatment Group 2 (2) n=10	3.50 (3.75)	0.75 (1.39)	0.29 (0.76)	2.35 (2.79)	1.20 (1.48)	0.50 (1.08)	0.80 (1.48)

Figure 6. Observed mean and standard deviations (SD) for the intensity of low back symptoms at the baseline and during the intervention and no-intervention periods.

Subgroups were formed at the individual level, the criteria being shoulder symptoms which to some degree had restricted participation in daily activities during the 12-month period preceding the intervention (n=34). The active component of the intervention, light resistance training, resulted in early significantly (p=0.050) reduced intensity of symptoms in the shoulder. The average estimated reduction in shoulder symptoms was calculated from the regression coefficient: -0.00222 (95% CI -0.00001696, -0.00442304). The regression coefficient indicates the reduction in symptoms if one minute is added to the training time during a given 5-week period. During the 5-week period, the average reduction in low back symptoms was 0.16 CR10 (95% CI 0.00-0.54) when the average training time during the 5-week period was 122 minutes (24 minutes per week, 5 minutes per working day). The intervention, ignoring the time spent performing light resistance training, did not have a significant effect on the intensity of low back symptoms.

According to the 0.27 CR10 value, in Treatment Group 1 the average estimated reduction was 10% (95% CI 0, 20) compared to the baseline measurement (2.7/CR10). In Treatment Group 2, it was 11% (95% CI 0, 23) compared to the last no-intervention measurement

(1.7/CR10). Figure 7 presents the observed mean and standard deviations (SD) for the intensity of shoulder symptoms at the baseline and during the intervention and no-intervention periods.

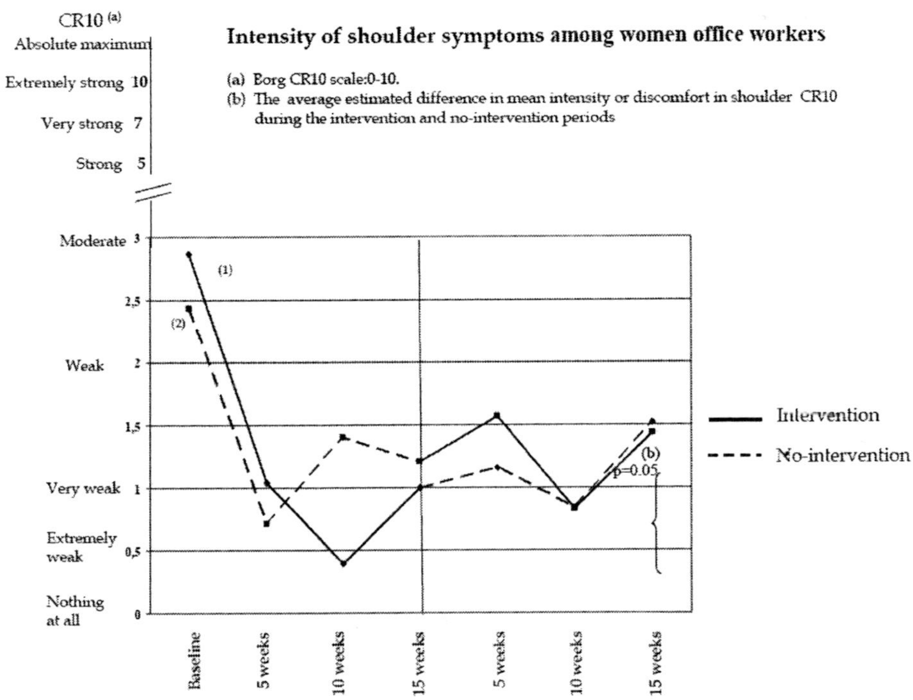

Observed mean (SD) of shoulder symptoms

	Baseline	Intervention			No-intervention		
Treatment Group 1 (1)	2.87 (2.32)	1.04 (1.85)	0.39 (0.72)	1.00 (1.73)	1.16 (1.46)	0.84 (1.73)	1.52 (2.04)
n=27	Baseline	No-intervention			Intervention		
Treatment Group 2 (2)	2.43 (2.24)	0.71 (1.25)	1.40 (1.95)	1.21 (1.15)	1.57 (1.51)	0.83 (1.33)	1.43 (1.81)
n=7							

Figure 7. Observed mean and standard deviations (SD) for the intensity of shoulder symptoms at the baseline and during the intervention and no-intervention periods.

Effects of Workplace Physical Exercise Intervention on Self-Confidence and Anxiety

The physical exercise intervention had no effect on somatic symptoms or mood in the whole women study group (n=68).

3.2.2. Effectiveness of a CRT Workplace Physical Exercise Intervention on Activities

Effects of Workplace Physical Exercise Intervention on Somatic Symptoms, Mood, Subjective Physical Well-Being and Subjective Physical Condition

The active component of the present intervention, light resistance training, significantly increased (p=0.016) subjective physical well-being. The average estimated increase in subjective physical well-being was calculated from the regression coefficient: 0.04370 (95% CI 0.0088316, 0.0785684). The regression coefficient indicates the increase in subjective physical well-being if one minute is added to the training time during a given 5-week period. During the 5-week intervention period, the average increase in subjective physical well-being was 5 units (95% CI 1, 10) when the average training time was 122 minutes (24 minutes per week, 5 minutes per working day).

According to the 5 units, in Treatment Group 1 the average estimated increase was 7% (95% CI 7, 14) compared to the baseline measurement (74 units). In Treatment Group 2, it was 6% (95% CI 1, 12) compared to the no-intervention measurement (80 units). Figure 8 presents the observed mean changes and 95% confidence intervals in subjective physical well-being between the treatment groups during the intervention and no-intervention periods.

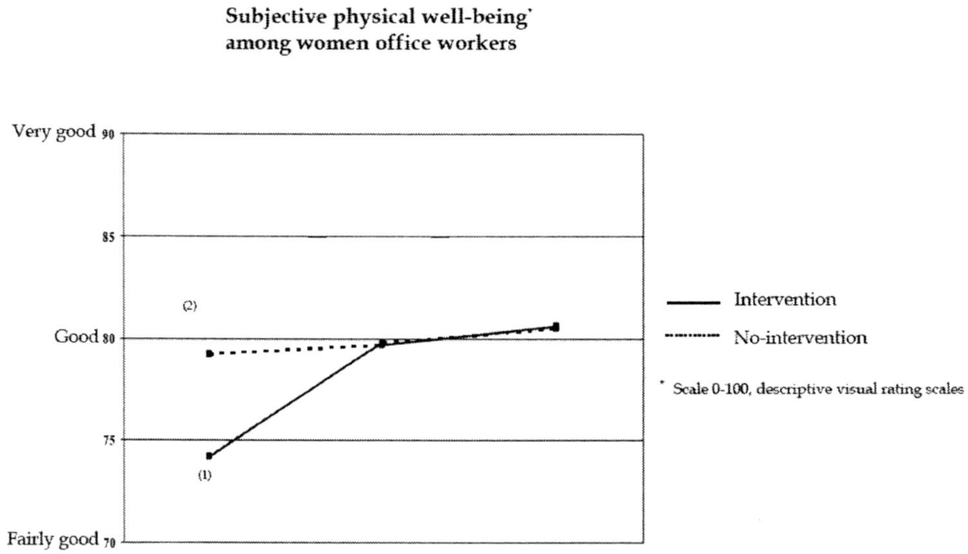

Observed mean (SD)

	Baseline	**Intervention**	No-intervention
Treatment Group 1 (1) -n=46	74.2 (14.0)	79.8 (14.1)	80.5 (12.7)
	Baseline	No-intervention	**Intervention**
Treatment Group 2 (2) -n=22	79.2 (13.2)	79.7 (15.4)	80.6 (11.4)

Figure 8. Observed mean changes and 95% confidence intervals in subjective physical well-being between the treatment groups during the intervention and no-intervention periods.

The active component of the present intervention, light resistance training, significantly increased (p=0.003) subjective physical condition (figure x). The average estimated increase in subjective physical condition was calculated from the regression coefficient: 0.05038 (95% CI 0.0179224, 0.0828376). The regression coefficient indicates the increase in subjective physical condition if one minute is added to the training time during a given 5-week period. During the 5-week intervention period, the average increase in subjective physical well-being was 6 units (95% CI 2, 10) when the average training time was 122 minutes (24 minutes per week, 5 minutes per working day).

According to the 6 units, in Treatment Group 1 the average estimated increase was 10% (95% CI 3, 17) compared to the baseline measurement (60 units). In Treatment Group 2, it was 11% (95% CI 4, 18) compared to the no-intervention measurement (56 units). Figure 9 presents the observed mean changes in subjective physical condition between the treatment groups at the baseline and during the intervention and no-intervention periods.

The physical exercise intervention had no effect on somatic symptoms or mood.

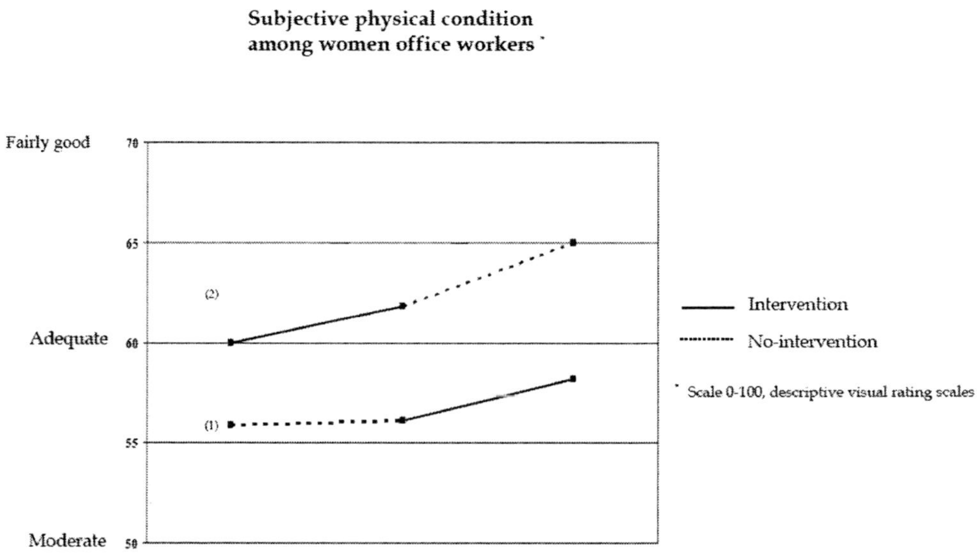

Observed mean (SD)

	Baseline	**Intervention**	No-intervention
Treatment Group 1 (1) -n=46	60.0 (14.4)	61.8 (15.1)	65.0 (14.3)
	Baseline	No-intervention	**Intervention**
Treatment Group 2 (2) -n=22	55.9 (15.9)	56.1 (20.5)	58.2 (17.9)

Figure 9. Observed mean changes in subjective physical condition between the treatment groups at the baseline and during the intervention and no-intervention periods.

3.2.3. Effectiveness of a CRT Workplace Physical Exercise Intervention on and Participation, Environmental Factors and General Subjective Well-Being

The active component of the present intervention, light resistance training, significantly increased (p=0.045) subjective working ability (figure x). The average estimated increase in subjective working ability was calculated from the regression coefficient: 0.02276 (95% CI 0.0007688, 0.0447512). The regression coefficient indicates the increase in subjective working ability if one minute is added to the training time during a given 5-week period. During the 5-week intervention period, the average increase in subjective working ability was 3 units (95% CI 1, 5) when the average training time was 122 minutes (24 minutes per week, 5 minutes per working day).

According to the 6 units, in Treatment Group 1 and 2 the average estimated increase was 3% (95% CI 1, 6) compared to the baseline or to the no-intervention measurement (87 units). Figure 10 presents the observed mean changes in subjective working ability between the treatment groups at the baseline and during the intervention and no-intervention periods.

The physical exercise intervention had no effect on mental stress at work, work atmosphere, life satisfaction or meaning of life.

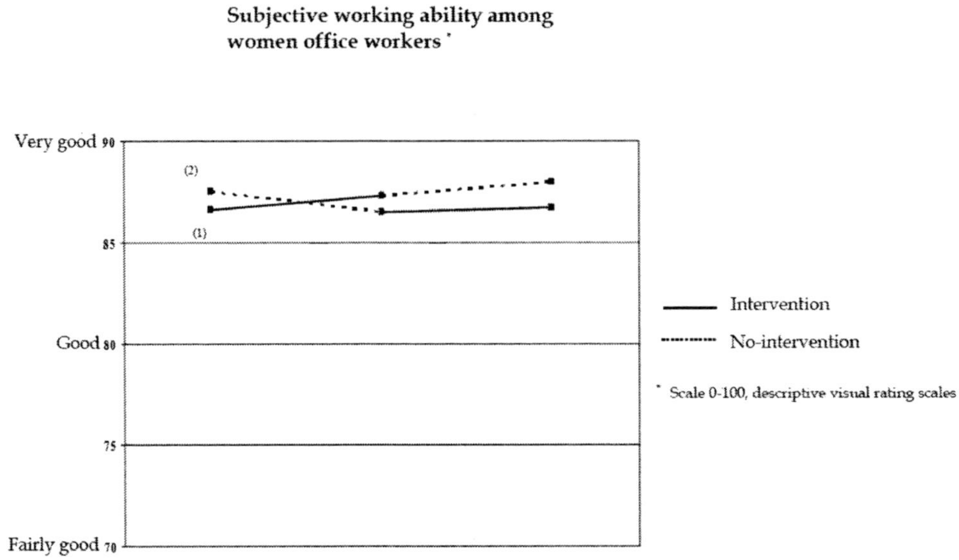

	Observed mean (SD)		
	Baseline	**Intervention**	No-intervention
Treatment Group 1 (1) -n=46	86.6 (11.2)	87.3 (11.4)	88.0 (9.3)
	Baseline	No-intervention	**Intervention**
Treatment Group 2 (2) -n=22	87.5 (7.5)	86.5 (9.0)	86.7 (5.6)

Figure 10. Observed mean changes in subjective working ability between the treatment groups at the baseline and during the intervention and no-intervention periods.

3.3. Controlling for Confounding Factors

Clustering and carry over effects: We found no clustering effects of workplace in our data as all the random department effects were non-significant; that is, department effects, the effects of individuals within departments, as well as their (random) interactions with the fixed factors. As the effect of the physical exercise intervention was similar in all four departments, we were able to simplify the original hierarchical model by leaving the department level out of the model. In cross-over designs, the results of the latter intervention period may be contaminated by some transference from the earlier period. According to the statistical analyses, there were no carry-over effects in the intensity of symptoms, or psychosocial measurements.

Learning and seasonal effects: We assumed that in this study population learning effects did not play a significant role in the intensity of symptoms or in the psychosocial or work ability measurements, because the main effect of the measurements was statistically significant only in low back pain measurements ($p=0.008$). There were no seasonal effects in our data, because no statistically significant differences in the intensity symptoms or psychosocial measurements between these two seasonal periods were found.

4. Discussion

4.1. Methodological Quality of CRT Study

The methodological quality of the CRT study, which were assessed according to the Physiotherapy evidence database (PEDro) quality score and Cochrane Collaboration criteria (van Tulder et al. 1997a, van Tulder et al. 1997b, Koes and Hovin 1998, Maher 2000), were high (PEDro 8/10). The methodological quality was lowered by the fact that neither the subjects nor the therapists were blinded. In physical exercise studies, it is very difficult or even impossible to blind subjects by including a placebo treatment, because it is not easy to develop a good and trustworthy placebo (Ojanen 1994, Shephard 1996, Koes and Hoving 1998, van Tulder et al. 2000, Liddle et al. 2004). In physical exercise interventions, in particular, the subjects cannot be made unaware that they have received treatment. Therefore, we maintain that physical exercise studies always include some non-specific effects, attraction or placebo effects. In the study we investigated the effect of the physical exercise intervention on the intensity of headache and neck, shoulder and low back symptoms among the women study population subgroups. The inclusion criteria in these two studies were determined after the physical exercise intervention. This kind of allocation, in practice, resulted in a more blinded study design, because neither subjects nor therapist knew who was included in the studied subgroup. In the standard cross-over design the order of the interventions is randomized for each cluster and a time period (called the "washout" period) is often allowed between the two interventions so that the first intervention does not affect the second. In our study we did not have a washout period between the two treatment periods, but we analysed the carry-over effects. If there were signs of carry-overs the results were analysed according to the first treatment period.

The strengths of our physical exercise intervention study were the randomisation by clusters in the natural working environment, controlling for possible confounding factors, such as department, learning, and seasonal effects, other physical activity (Guyatt et al. 1993, Liddle et al. 2004), and careful documentation of the training dose (Hide and Bø, 1998). Total PA, including OPA, commuting, LTPA and the physical exercise intervention should be determined to a sufficient level of accuracy, for instance according to METs (Mälkiä et al. 1994, Mälkiä 1996, ACSM 1998, ACSM 2000, Howley 2001, Kesäniemi et al. 2001). Moreover, a cross-over trial is ethically more acceptable and statistically more efficient than similar-sized parallel group trials.

The intention-to-treat approach is often inadequately described and inadequately applied. Authors should describe the handling of deviations from randomised allocations and missing responses and discuss the potential effect of any missing response (Hollis and Campbell 1999). The absence of an intention-to-treat analysis in intervention studies can lead to a bias since subjects may drop out because for reasons that make them non comparable with the group that completes the study with respect to the outcome variable. If the intention-to-treat analysis is not performed the effectiveness of treatment may be overestimated (Proper 2002). In their critical review Proper et al. (2002) found that only one out of eight workplace intervention studies had included an intention-to-treat analysis, and this study was a controlled trial. In our CRT cross-over study the intention-to-treat analysis meant that all subjects, who were randomly assigned to the two treatment sequence groups (Treatment

Group 1 and Treatment Group 2), were analysed together, regardless of whether or not they completed or received the physical exercise intervention treatment. An advantage of mixed models (Brown and Prescott 1999, Goldstein 1995), compared to ANOVA (or MANOVA) for repeated measures, is that there is no technical need to exclude subjects with incomplete data from the analysis. Instead, all the available observations, whether from completers or non-completers, contribute to the statistical inference (parameter estimation, significance testing) by virtue of the likelihood-based estimation method. In the mixed model approach we assume that each single observation obeys the same specified model, even where the observation is lacking no matter if it is observed or not. The model compensates for the missing data. The validity of this model assumption (and inference) requires, however, that the possible drop-out mechanism is random. In our study the number of non-completers was small and we can assume that the drop-out were random. Thus we do not see any problems of bias due to the incompleteness of the data.

4.2. Results of the CRT Study

Our originally study reports among women and men office workers study population indicated that the physical exercise intervention degreased intensity of headache, and neck and low back symptoms (Sjögren et al 2005, Sjögren et al 2006a). Among women office workers, in addition, the light resistance training degreased almost statistically significantly the intensity of shoulder symptoms. Our previous study findings and also this study finding among women support those of the previous studies according to which workplace-based physical exercise interventions can reduce musculoskeletal symptoms (Griffiths 1996, Linton and van Tulder 2001, Maher 2000, Proper et al. 2003, van Poppel et al. 2004, Tveito et al. 2004). However, our subgroup analyze among women did not degrease the intensity of musculoskeletal symptoms more than in our originally study population thought women baseline measurements in physical psychosocial functioning and work ability were lower level than men. The baseline difference between women and men obviously was not enough to show clearer intervention effect. Regardless the frequency, duration and intensity of the light resistance training and guidance observed in the workplace in our study, seems to be adequate to alleviate musculoskeletal symptoms, although the dose was lower than we recommended also among women. Adherence rates, like numbers of training sessions and training times in minutes did not differ by gender.

We found a statistically significant correspondence between light resistance training and increased subjective physical well-being, subjective physical condition and subjective working ability, but not between training and the other psychosocial functioning, like anxiety, mood and self-confidence, mental stress of work, working atmosphere or general well-being variables studied. In the other words, our study supports the findings of previous studies that the effect of physical exercise interventions in the workplace on psychosocial functioning among healthy middle age populations is inconclusive (Griffiths 1996, Proper et al. 2003) also among subgroup of women. The meagre results obtained on psychosocial functioning in our study are probably due to the ceiling effect, as the subjects were middle-aged healthy volunteers whose level of psychosocial functioning and general subjective well-being was already high at the baseline, thought physical and psychosocial functioning were worse among women than men at the baseline. Hence there is still also a need to study the effectiveness of exercise on psychosocial functioning and general well-being in larger populations with a clearer lower baseline level of well-being. However, our results were not entirely unequivocal, as the active component of the intervention, light resistant training, increased the subjective physical well-being and subjective work ability of the women office workers studied, despite their high baseline values.

The efficacy of the physical exercise intervention on musculoskeletal symptoms and subjective physical well-being might be more due to training specificity, because the estimated MET hours of light exercise training and its percentage of LTPA (average 8.7%) and AT MET hours (average 1.5%) were on a low-level, as can be seen in figure x. Because the percentage proportion of LTPA were higher among women than men (5.7%) , the it would be important to have also follow-up studies of long duration to explore the possibility that higher proportion of LTPA could improve women's physical and psychosocial prerequisites of functioning, work ability and general well-being better than men. The percentage proportion of OPA should be measured more carefully in the future studies. However according to the averages (1.5 MET of OPA, eight hours working days, 5-week period) the training METS was 9.7% of OPA, although the absolute time spent on training during the same time period was only 1%. Could this physical exercise intervention be enough cost-benefits or cost-effectiveness should be taken into account in further intervention studies.

The main idea behind our physical exercise intervention was to counterbalance sedentary work or to obtain relief from monotonous and fixed working positions. However, as a whole, the intervention also showed willingness by the employer to do something about the physical and psychosocial functioning and work ability of the employees and to enhance opportunities for organisational and fellow worker support. Our results show that the physical exercise intervention was successful especially in alleviating musculoskeletal symptoms. Changes in this component were important, as in our study Sjögren-Rönkä et al. 2002 we found that the intensity of musculoskeletal symptoms had the greatest negative effect on work ability. The next need following on from the physical exercise intervention would be an intervention targeted at improving job content and decreasing psychosocial pressure at work. We have recommend that the workplace studied the rehabilitation should be directed, first, at reducing musculoskeletal symptoms and improving physical condition, particularly in women and, second, at reducing mental stress at work and improving the working atmosphere (Sjögren-Rönkä et al. 2001). Also Fogelman and Lewis et al. (2002) successes that among VDT workers the main foci in reducing musculoskeletal symptoms are workstation ergonomics, the need to limit the number of uninterrupted hours at the keyboard and the psychosocial work environment. Other recommendations for ways to reduce the stress of human computer interaction at work have included proper ergonomic conditions, increased organisational support, improved job content, an appropriate workload to decrease pressure of work, and enhanced opportunities for social support (Smith et al. 1999).

Strazdins and Bammer (2004) found gender differences in risk factor among public service employees in Australia. At work, for example, women sat in the same position for long periods of time, worked longer days on a computer and had more repetitive movements than men. In addition, women spent considerably less time than men exercising or relaxing during leisure-time. Also in our study leisure time physical activity were lower among women than men at the baseline measurements; time-weighted intensity of leisure time was among women 3.6 MET and among men 5.6 MET, and maximum intensity of leisure time was among women, 4.3 MET and among men 6.9 MET (Sjögren 2006). Physical exercise interventions might be even more helpful in maintaining work ability and preventing impairment in work ability among women the than among men, particularly at older ages.

4.3. Clinical Importance and Generalization of the RCT Study Findings

The comparability of clinically important differences or changes between previous studies and our study is difficult because of different study populations, pain measurements and treatments. In previous intervention studies, clinically important positive changes from the subject's perspective, the changes in intensity of musculoskeletal symptoms (scales 0-10) have been defined on average among different patient populations as 30 percentual or to 2 absolute points (Farrar et al. 2000, Farrar et al. 2001, Hägg et al. 2003). The corresponding values among a rheumatoid arthritis patient population were 20% or 1.2 (Goldsmith et al. 1993). However in less disabled populations even small changes can be clinically important (Farrar et al. 2000, Farrar et al. 2001, Hägg et al. 2003). In the critical review by Proper et al. (2003) of workplace physical activity programs, health-related benefits were considered to have a positive effect where statistically significant results or a relevant effect size, determined as over 20% difference between study groups, were obtained. Among our healthy middle age women population the physical exercise intervention led to changes of 11-46 per cent or to absolute changes 0.3-0.6 CR0 in the intensity of musculoskeletal symptoms, and it led to changes of 3-11 per cent or absolute changes 3-6 units in the subjective functioning (physical well-being, condition and working ability). We can assume that our specific exercise was clinically important in alleviating the intensity of symptoms, especially headache and neck symptoms, but also in low back symptoms, but the results were only tentative on subjective functioning. Although, there was a low level of systematic error during the physical exercise intervention and follow-up study (selection bias, information bias, confounding factors), care must be taken in generalizing the study results beyond the target population (women office workers) as we were not able to control for all non-specific effects, and as the study samples were relatively small.

To confirm assumptions of the effectiveness of physical exercise interventions, more randomized and controlled follow-up studies among both gender, different sedentary occupations and workplaces are required. There is also a need to study the effects of different training doses and movements, using different training tools and methods of guidance, to clarify the role of PA for physical and psychosocial functioning. Follow-up studies of long duration are also needed to explore the possibility that even slight positive changes could be important in preventing impairments in people's physical and psychosocial prerequisites of functioning, work ability and general well-being.

References

American College of Sports Medicine (ACSM). 1998. The recommended quantity and quality of exercise for developing and maintaining cardiorespiratory and muscular fitness and flexibility in healthy adults. *Medicine and Science in Sports and Exercise.* 30, 975-991.

American College of Sports Medicine (ACSM). 2000. *Guidelines for exercise testing and prescription,* 6th edn. Philadelphia: Lippincott Williams and Wilkins.

Andersson K, Karlenhagen S, Jonsson B. 1987. The importance of variations in questionnaire administration. *Applied Ergomics.* 18.3, 229-232.

Baker NA, Jacobs K, Tickle-Degnen. 2003. The association between the meaning of working and musculoskeletal discomfort. *International Journal of Industrial Ergonomics.* 31, 235-247.

Bergqvist U, Wolgast E, Nilsson B, Voss M. 1995. Musculoskeletal disorders among visual display terminal workers: individual, ergonomic, and work organizational factors. *Ergonomics.* 38(4), 763-776.

Borg G. 1998. Borg's perceived exertion and pain scales, Champaign (IL): Human Kinetics.

Bovim G, Schrader H, Sand T. 1994. Neck pain in the general population. *Spine.* 19(12), 1307-1309.

Braith RW, Graves JE, Leggett SH, Pollock ML.1993. Effect of training on the relationship between maximal and submaximal strength. *Medicine and Science in Sports and Exercise.* 25, 132-138.

Brown H, Prescott R. 1999. *Applied Mixed Models in Medicine.* Chichester: John Wiley and Sons, 202.

Campbell MK, Elbourne DR, Altman DG. 2004. Consort statement: extension to cluster randomized trials. *British Medical Journal.* 328, 702-708.

Dishman RK, Oldenburg B, O'Neal H, Shephard RJ. 1998. Worksite physical activity interventions. *American Journal of Preventive Medicine.* 15(4), 344-361.

Dworkin RH, Turk DC, Farrar JT, Haythornthwaite JA, Jensen MP, Katz NP, Kerns RD, Stucki G,Allen RR, Bellamy N, Carr DB, Chandler J, Cowan P, Dionne R, Galer BS, Hertz S, Jadad R, Kramer LD, Manning DC, Martin S, McCormick CG, McDermott MP, McGrath P, Quessy S, Rappaport BA, Robbins W, Robinson JP, Rothman M, Royal MA, Simon L, Stauffer JW, Stain W, Tollett J, Wernicke J, Witter J. 2005. Topical review and recommendations. Core outcome measures for chronic pain clinical trials: IMMPACT recommendations. *Pain.* 113, 9-19.

Ekberg K, Karlsson M, Axelson O, Axelson, Björkqvist B, Bjerre-Kiely B, Malm P. 1995. Cross-sectional study of risk factors for symptoms in the neck and shoulder area. *Ergonomics.* 38(5), 971-980.

Eriksen HR, Svensrød R, Ursin G, Ursin H. 1998. Pevalence of subjective health complaints in the Nordic European countries in 1993. *European Journal of Public Health.* 8, 294-298.

Farrar JT, Portenoy RK, Berlin JA, Kinman JL, Strom BL. 2000. Defining the clinically important difference in pain outcome measures. *Pain.* 88, 287-94.

Farrar JT, Young Jr. JP, LaMoreaux L, Werth JL, Poole RM. 2001. Clinical importance of changes in chronic pain intensity measured on an 11-point numerical pain rating scale. Pain 94, 149-58.

Fogleman M, Lewis RJ. 2002. Factors associated with self-reported musculoskeletal discomfort in video display terminal (VDT) user. *International Journal of Industrial Ergonomics.* 29, 311-318.

Forsman M, Taoda K, Thorn S, Zhang Q. 2002. Motor-unit recruitment during long-term isometric and wrist motion contractions: a study concerning muscular pain development in computer operators. *International Journal of Industrial Ergonomics.* 30, 237-250.

Fredriksson K, Alfredsson L, Thorbjörnsson CB, Punnett L, Toomingas A, Torgén M, Kiblom Å. 2000. Risk factors for neck and shoulder disorders: A nested case-control study covering a 24-year period. American Journal of Industrial Medicine 38, 516-528.

Goldsmith CH, Boers M, Bombardier C, Tugwell P. 1993. Criteria for clinically important changes in outcomes: development, scoring and evaluation of rheumatoid arthritis patents and trial profiles. *Journal of Rheumatology.* 20, 561-565.

Goldstein H. 1995. *Multilevel statistical models.* Second edition. London: Arnold, 50,70.

Griffiths A. 1996. The benefits of employee exercise programmes: a review. *Work and Stress.* 10(1), 5-23.

Guyatt GH, Sackett DL, Cook DJ. 1993. Users' guides to the medical literature. II. How to use an article about therapy or prevention. A. Are the results of the study valid? *Journal of the American Medical Association.* 1, 2598-2601.

Hakkanen M, Viikari-Juntura E, Martikainen R. 2001. Job experience, work load, and risk of musculoskeletal disorder. *Occupational and Environmental Medicine.* 58(2), 129-135.

Hales TR, Sauter SL, Peterson MR, Fine LJ, Putz-Anderson V, Schleifer LR, Ochs TT, Bernard BP. 1994. Musculoskeltal disorders among visual display terminals users in telecommunicatios company. *Egonomics.* 37(10), 1603-1621.

Hellsing AL, Bryngelsson IL. 2000. Predictors of musculoskeletal pain in men: A twenty-year follow-up from examination at enlistment. *Spine.* 25(23), 3080-3086.

Hide G, Bø K. 1998. Effect of exercise in the treatment of chronic low back pain: a systematic review, emphasising type and dose of exercise. *Physical therapy reviews.* 3, 107-117.

Hollis S, Campbell F. 1999. What is meant by intention to treat analysis? Survey of published randomized controlled trials. *British Medical Journal.* 319, 670-674.

Hoogendoorn WE, van Poppel MNM, Bongers PM, Koes BW, Bouter LM. 2000a. Systematic review of psychosocial factors at work and private life as risk factors for back pain. *Spine.* 25(16), 2114-2125.

Howley ET. 2001. Type of activity: resistance, aerobic and leisure versus occupational activity. *Medicine and Science in Sport and Medicine.* 33(6), S364-S369.

Hägg O, Fritzell P, Nordwall A. 2003. The clinical importance of changes in outcome scores after treatment for chronic low back pain. *European Spine Journal.* 12, 12-20.

Ilmarinen J. 1999. Ageing workers in the European Union – Status and promotion of work ability, employability and employment. Finnish Institute of Occupational Health, Ministry of Social Affairs and Health, Ministry of Labour. Painotalo Miktor Ky, Helsinki, Finland.

ISO/FDIS 8996. 2004. Ergonomics of thermal environment – determination of metabolic rate. Final draft.

Kaikkonen H, Yrjämä M, Siljander E, Byman P, Laukkanen R. 2000. The effect of heart rate controlled low resistance circuit weight training and edurance training on maximal aerobic power in sedentary adults. Skandinavian. *Journal of Medicine and Science in Sport.* 10, 211-215.

Kansanterveys laitos (KTL). 2004. Health and functional capacity in Finland. Baseline results of the health 2000 health examination survey (Aromaa A, Koskinen S, editors). KTL-National Public Health Institute, Finland. Department of Health and Functional Capacity. Helsinki 2004.

Koes BW, Hoving JL. 1998. The value of the randomized clinical trial in the field of physiotherapy. *Manual Therapy.* 3(4), 179-86.

Kesäniemi YA, Danforth E JR., Jensen MD, PG Kopelman, Lefebvre P, Reeder BA. 2001. Dose-response issues concerning physical activity and health: an evidence-based symposium. *Medicine and Science in sports and Exercise.* 3(suppl), 351-358.

Kuorinka I, Jonsson B, Kiblom A, Vinterberg H, Biering-Sørensen F, Andersson G, et al. 1987. Standardised Nordic questionnaires for the analysis of musculoskeletal symptoms. *Applied Ergonomics.* 18.3, 223-237.

Liddle SD, Baxter GD, Gracey JH. 2004. Exercise and chronic low back pain: what works? *Pain.* 107, 176-90.

Linton SL. 2000. A review of psychological risk factors in back and neck pain. *Spine.* 25(9), 1148-1156.

Linton SJ, Kamwendo K. 1989.Risk factors in the physical work environment for neck and shoulder pain in secretaries. *Journal of Occupational Medicine.* 31(7), 609-613.

Linton SJ, van Tulder MW. 2001. Preventive interventions for back and neck pain problems: what is the evidence? *Spine.* 26(7), 778-787.

Luoma K, Riihimäki H, Luukkonen R, Raininko R, Viikari-Juntura E, Lamminen A. 2000. Low back pain in relation to lumbar disc degeneration. *Spine.* 25(4), 487-492.

Maher CG, 2000. A systematic review of workplace interventions to prevent low back pain. *Australian Journal of Physiotherapy.* 46, 259-69.

McDonagh MJ, Daves CT. 1984.Adaptive response of mammalian skeletal muscle to exercise with high loads. *European Journal of Applied Physiology.* 52, 139-155.

Mäkelä M, Heliövaara M, Sievers K, Impivaara O, Aromaa A. 1991. Prevalence determinants, and consequences of chronic neck pain in Finland. *American Journal of Epidemiology.* 134(11), 1356-1367.

Mälkiä E, Impivaara O, Heliövaara M, Maatela J. 1994. The physical activity of healthy and chronically ill adults in Finland at work, at leisure, and during commuting. *Scandinavian Journal of Medicine and Science in Sports.* 4, 82-87.

Mälkiä E. 1996. MET based questionnaire for the study of physical activity. In: Mälkiä E, Sihvonen S, editors. *Assessment of function and movement.* Selected papers. Third Nordic symposium on physiotherapy. Jyväskylä: PainoPorras oy, 91-103.

Ojanen, M. 1994. Physical exercise and psychological well-being The Finnish Society for *Research in Sport and Physical Education,* Report no 19, Helsinki (in Finnish) 1994.

Ojanen M. 2000. Effects of illness and adversity on quality of life. In: Jobin J, Maltais F, Le Blanc P, Simard C, eds. *Advances in cardiopulmonary rehabilitation,* Champaign IL: Human Kinetics Press, 198-210.

Patterson HD, Thompson R. 1971. Recovery of inter-block information when block-sizes are unequal. *Biometrika.* 58, 545-554.

Pope DP, Croft PR, Pritchard CM, Siman AJ, Macfarlane GJ. 1997. Occupational factors related to shoulder pain and disability. *Occupational and Environmental Medicine.* 54, 316-321.

Proper KI, Staal BJ, Hildebrand VH, van der Beek AJ, van Mechelen W. 2002. Effectiveness of physical activity programs at worksites with respect to work-related outcomes. *Scandinavian Journal of Work, Environment and Health.* 28(2), 75-84.

Proper K, Koning M, van der Beek A, Hildebrant VH, Bosscher RJ, van Mechelen W. 2003. The effectiveness of worksite physical activity programs on physical activity, physical fitness, and health. *Clinical Journal of Sport Medicine.* 13, 106-17

Rönkä T, Kaikkonen H, Virtanen P, Laukkanen R, Mälkiä E. 2000.

Cardiovascular response during one light resistance training exercise session.5th Annual Congress of the European College of Sport Science. Jyväskylä 2000, Finland. Proceedings, 635.

Sakamoto Y, Ishiguro M, Kitagawa G. 1986. Akaike information criterion statistics. Dordrecht: Reidel.

SAS. SAS/STAT User's Guide. 1999. Version 8. Volume 2. Cary, NC: SAS Institute Inc.

Schmidt, R. A. 1991. Motor Learning and Performance. From principles to practice. University of California, Los Angeles. Human Kinetics Books. Champaign, Illinois.

Seistamo J, Klockars M. 1997. Aging and changes in health. *Scandinavian Journal of Work Environment and Health.* 23(suppl 1), 27-35.

Shephard RJ. 1996. Worksite fitness and exercise programs: A review of methodology and health impact. *American Journal of Health Promotion.* 10(6), 436-452.

Sibbald B, Roberts C. 1998. Understanding controlled trials Crossover trials. British Medical Journal 316, 1719-1720.

Sjögren T. 2006. Effectiveness of a workplace physical exercise intervention on the functioning, work ability, and subjective well-being of office workers – a cluster randomised controlled cross-over trial with one-year follow-up. Jyväskylä: University of Jyväskylä, 2006, 99 p.(*Studies in Sport, Physical Education and Health,* ISSN 0356-1070; 118) ISBN 951-39-2518-8

Sjögren T, Nissinen K, Järvenpää S, Ojanen M, Vanharanta, H, Mälkiä E. 2005. Effects of a workplace physical exercise intervention on the intensity of headache and neck and shoulder symptoms and upper extremity muscular strength of office workers: A cluster randomized controlled cross-over trial. *Pain.* 116, 119-128.

Sjögren T, Nissinen K, Järvenpää S, Ojanen M, Vanharanta H, Mälkiä E. 2006a. Effects of workplace physical exercise intervention on the intensity of low back symptoms of office workers: A cluster randomized controlled cross-over design. *Journal of Back and Musculoskeletal Rehabilitation.* 19, 13-24.

Sjögren T, Nissinen K, Järvenpää S, Ojanen M, Vanharanta H, Mälkiä E.2006b. Effects of a physical exercise intervention on the subjective well-being, psychosocial functioning and general well-being among office workers: A cluster randomized controlled cross-over design.*Scandinavian Journal of Medicine and Science in Sports.* 16,381-390.

Sjögren-Rönkä T, Ojanen M, Mustalampi S, Mälkiä E. 2001. Musculoskeletal symptoms and psychosocial functioning by gender and age on subjects with sedentary occupation. NES 2001 Nordic Ergonomics Society 33 rd Annual Congress. *Promotion of Health through Ergonomic Working and Living Conditions. Outcomes and methods of research and practice.* Tampere, Finland. Proceedings, p. 422.

Sjögren-Rönkä T, Ojanen MT, Leskinen EK, Mustalampi ST, Mälkiä EA. 2002.Physical and psychosocial prerequisites of functioning in relation to work ability and general subjective well-being among office workers. *Scandinavian Journal of Work Environ and Health.* 28(3),184-190.

Smith MJ, Conway FT, Karsh BT. 1999. Occupational stress in human computer interaction. Industrial Health 37(2), 157-173.

STM, Ministry of Social Affairs and Health. 2004. *Trends in social protection.* 1998-1999. Publication of the Ministry of Social Affairs and Health, eng.

Strazdins L, Bammer G. 2004. Women, work and musculoskeletal health. Social Science and Medicine 58, 997-1005.

Thorbjornsson CB, Alfredsson L, Fredriksson K, Michelsén H, Punnett L, Vingård E., Torgén M, Kilbom Å. 2000. Physical and psychosocial factors related to low back pain during 24-year period. A nested case-control analysis. *Spine.* 25(3), 369-374.

Tola S, Riihimäki H, Videman T, Viikari-Juntura E, Hänninen K. 1988. Neck and shoulder symptoms among men in machine operating, dynamic physical work and sedentary work. *Scandinavian journal of work environment and health.* 14, 299-305.

Työterveyslaitos (TTL). *Work and health survey.* 2000. Charts and tables. Finnish Institute of Occupational Health. Helsinki (in Finnish).

Työterveyslaitos (TTL). *Work and health survey.* 2003. Charts and tables. Finnish Institute of Occupational Health. Helsinki (in Finnish).

Turk DC, Dworkin RH, Allen RR, Bellamy N, Brandenburg N, Carr DB, Cleeland C, Dionne R, Farrar JT, Galer BS, Hewitt DJ, Jadad A, Katz NP, Kramer LD, Manning DC, McCormick CG, McDermott M, McGrath P, Quessy S, Rappaport BA, Robinson JP, Royal MA, Simon L, Stauffer JW, Stein W, Tollett J, Witter J. 2003. Core outcome domains for chronic pain clinical trials: IMMPACT recommendations. *Pain.* 106, 337-345.

Tveito TH, Hysing M, Eriksen HR. 2004. Low back pain interventions at the workplace: a systematic literature review. *Occupational Medicine.* 54(1), 3-13.

van Tulder MW, Assendelft JJ, Koes BW, Bouter LM. 1997a. Method guidelines for systematic reviews in the Cochrane Collaboration Back Review Group for spinal disorders. *Spine.* 22(20), 2323-2330.

van Tulder MW, Koes BW, Bouter LM. 1997b. Conservative treatment of acute and chronic nonspecific back pain: a systematic review of randomized controlled trials of the most common interventions. *Spine.* 22(18), 2128-2156.

van Tulder M, Malmivaara A, Esmail R. 2000. Exercise therapy for loeb back pain. Asystematic review within the framework of Cochrane Colloboration Back Revieew Group. *Spine.* 25(21), 2784-2796.

Viikari-Juntura E, Martikainen R, Luukkonen R, Mutanen P, Takala EP, Riihimäki H. 2001. Longitudinal study on work-related and individual risk factors affecting radiating neck pain. *Occupational and Environmental Medicine.* 58(5), 345-352.

WHO. ICF/ICIDH-2. 2001. International classification of functioning, disability and health. Final draft, full version. Classification, assessment, surveys, and terminology team. World Health Organization. Geneva, Switzerland. http:/www.who.int/icidh

In: Exercise and Women's Health
Editor: Laura A. Charlington, pp. 99-112
ISBN: 978-1-60456-013-8

Chapter 4

PAIN AND PHYSICAL ACTIVITY IN WOMEN WITH MS: DIFFERENTIAL PATTERN OF RELATIONSHIPS WITH OBJECTIVE AND SELF-REPORT MEASURES OF PHYSICAL ACTIVITY

Erin M. Snook*[1], *Rachael C. Gliottoni*[1], *Robert W. Motl*[*1], *Dane B. Cook*[2] and *Patrick J. O'Connor*[3]

[1] University of Illinois at Urbana-Champaign
[2] William S. Middleton Memorial Veterans Hospital
and University of Wisconsin at Madison
[3] University of Georgia

ABSTRACT

Multiple sclerosis (MS) is a common neurological disease that primarily affects adult Caucasian women. Pain is a frequently reported symptom associated with MS with prevalence estimates ranging from 29% to 90% of patients. The pain associated with MS can interfere with activities of daily living and result in disability, and might be a barrier for participation in physical activity. Accordingly, pain might serve as a partial explanation for the predominance of physical inactivity in persons with MS. This study involved an examination of the relationships between several aspects of pain and self-report and objective measures of physical activity in two independent samples of women with MS (*N*s = 88 and 28). The women in both samples completed the Short-form of the McGill Pain Questionnaire (SF-MPQ) and then wore an accelerometer for seven days and completed the Godin Leisure-Time Exercise Questionnaire (GLTEQ). The SF-MPQ consists of 15 descriptors that yield sensory (SF-MPQS; sensory quality of pain), affective (SF-MPQA; affective qualities of pain), and overall or total (SF-MPQT) pain quality ratings. The SF-MPQ contains an additional item that measures the overall intensity of pain or Present Pain Index (PPI). We conducted Pearson product-moment

* Address all correspondence to Robert W. Motl, Ph.D., Department of Kinesiology and Community Health, University of Illinois, 350 Freer Hall, Urbana, IL 61801. Phone: (217) 265-0886. Fax: (217) 333-3124. Electronic Mail: robmotl@uiuc.edu

correlations for examining the relationships between scores on the SF-MPQ, accelerometer, and GLTEQ in the two independent samples separately. Within the first sample ($N = 88$), there were significant correlations between the SF-MPQT ($r = -.29$, $p = .01$), SF-MPQS ($r = -.22$, $p = .04$), SF-MPQA ($r = -.39$, $p = .001$), and PPI ($r = -.29$, $p = .01$) scores and accelerometer counts. Scores from the SF-MPQ were not significantly correlated ($p > .05$) with GLTEQ scores. Within the second sample ($N = 28$), there was a similar pattern of results such that SF-MPQT ($r = -.40$, $p = .02$), SF-MPQS ($r = -.40$, $p = .02$), SF-MPQA ($r = -.30$, $p = .05$), and PPI ($r = -.45$, $p = .01$) scores from the SF-MPQ were significantly correlated with accelerometer counts. Again, scores from the SF-MPQ were not significantly correlated ($p > .05$) with GLTEQ scores. The observed pattern of results indicates that sensory and affective dimensions of pain as well as the overall intensity of pain are associated with objectively measured physical activity in the two independent samples of individuals with MS. One potential implication is that pain does play a role in physical activity participation, but the relationship is not immediately recognized by participants based on the lack of relationships with the self-report measurement of physical activity.

INTRODUCTION

Multiple sclerosis (MS) affects approximately 2.5 million people world wide, including an estimated 400,000 Americans (National Multiple Sclerosis Society [NMSS], 2005). MS is most commonly diagnosed in adult Caucasian women between 20 – 50 years of age. Indeed, MS is two to three times more prevalent among women than men and is more common among individuals of northern European descent than people of African, Asian, and Hispanic ancestry (NMSS, 2005).

MS is a chronic neurological disease that involves intermittent bursts of focal inflammation in the central nervous system (CNS) leading to demyelination and transection of axons in the brain, optic nerves, and spinal cord. The demyelination and transection of axons block or delay the conduction of electrical potentials along axonal pathways in the CNS. This interference with neuronal conduction is associated with pain and other symptoms experienced by people with MS (Lublin, 2005; Schapiro, 2003).

Pain, "an unpleasant sensory or emotional experience associated with actual or potential tissue damage or described in terms of such damage" (International Associations for the Study of Pain [IASP], 1979, p. 249), is a common symptom experienced by individuals with MS (Crayton and Rossman, 2006). The prevalence of pain in MS has ranged from 29 - 90% (Clifford and Trotter, 1984; Kalia and O'Connor, 2005), with the majority of pain prevalence rates ranging between 43 - 80% (e.g., Ehde, Osborne, and Jensen, 2005; Solaro, et al., 2004; Stenager, Knudsen, Jensen, 1991, 1995; Svendsen et al., 2003). For example, one recent large scale investigation of 10,176 patients from the NARCOMS Patient Registry found that 49% of respondents reported mild to severe pain during the previous month (Hadjimichael, Kerns, Rizzo, Cutter, and Vollmer, 2007).

There are other features that further characterize the pain experienced by individuals with MS. The pain can result from a primary lesion or dysfunction in the peripheral or central nervous system and can include dyesthetic pain (i.e., abnormal sensations such as burning) and neuralgia (Schapiro, 2003), or the pain can be felt in the bones, muscles, joints, and other body tissue (Solaro, Lunardi, and Mancardi, 2003). We further note that pain experienced by those with MS occurs in a variety of sites. One recent study of 180 individuals with MS identified 17 pain locations and pain most commonly occurred in the legs (75%), lower back (59%), and neck (52%; Ehde, Osborne, Hanley, Jensen, and Kraft, 2006). Another study reported that pain most commonly occurred in the legs, and the most common sensations were spasms, aching, and tingling or crawling (Hadjimichael et al., 2007).

The pain experienced by those with MS is associated with a variety of functional and behavioral outcomes, including reduced mobility and interference with daily activities (Hadjimichael et al., 2007; Svendsen, Jensen, Hansen, and Bach, 2005). For example, one recent study reported that pain interferes with mobility and recreational activities in individuals with MS (Ehde et al., 2006). Pain has been inversely and moderately associated with MS-related disability (e.g., $d = -.49$ for those experiencing severe pain versus those without pain), and negatively and strongly associated with perceived participation in recreational and work activities (e.g., $d = -.87$ for those experiencing mild, moderate, and severe pain versus those without pain) and one's ability to walk or move around (e.g., $d = -.75$ for those experiencing mild, moderate, and severe pain versus those without pain) (Hadjimichael et al., 2007). Moreover, one study has reported that pain interfered with daily activities more often among individuals with MS than in matched controls without MS (Svendsen et al., 2005).

Beyond mobility and daily activities, pain may be associated with reduced participation in physical activity among those with MS. Physical activity has been defined by Bouchard and Shephard (1994, p. 77) as "any body movement produced by the skeletal muscles that results in a substantial increase over the resting energy expenditure" and there is evidence that individuals with MS are less physically active than non-diseased individuals ($d = -.96$; Motl, McAuley, and Snook, 2005). There are several reasons that pain may be associated with reduced physical activity in MS. First, recent studies have demonstrated an inverse relationship between global MS-related symptoms and physical activity (Motl, Snook, McAuley, and Gliottoni, 2006; Motl et al., in press), although those studies did not focus on pain as a specific correlate of physical activity. Second, pain in MS is most commonly experienced in the legs, thereby providing a substantial sensory barrier for common types of physical activity such as walking, jogging, and cycling. Third, pain reported by MS patients is associated with functional and behavioral outcomes of reduced mobility and interference with daily activities, respectively (Hadjimichael et al., 2007; Svendsen et al., 2005).

Despite the aforementioned rationale, to our knowledge no published studies have directly examined the relationship between pain and physical activity in individuals with MS. Therefore, this study examined the relationship between pain symptoms and physical activity participation in two samples of individuals with MS. This relationship was examined in two samples that were recruited for different studies in order to provide independent evidence of an association between pain and physical activity. The first sample was participating in a study that did not focus on pain and physical activity, whereas the second sample was recruited for a study that focused on pain and physical activity in MS. Within both samples, we expected that pain would be significantly and negatively associated with physical activity as assessed by both self-report and objective measures of physical activity.

METHODOLOGY

Participants

Participants were recruited through the Greater Illinois and Indiana State Chapters of the National Multiple Sclerosis Society and demographic information for both samples are included in table 1. Sample 1 were participants recruited into a study of global and specific symptoms as correlates of physical activity in MS and the sample included 88 females with an average age of 51.0 (SD = 11.9) years. The sample was primarily Caucasian (n = 85, 96.6%), employed (n = 47, 53.4%), married (n = 65, 73.9%) and well educated (college graduate n = 43, 48.9%). The mean duration since MS diagnosis was 12.7 (SD = 9.6) years and there were 58 participants (65.9%), with relapsing-remitting MS, 26 (29.5%) with secondary progressive MS, one (1.1) with primary progressive and two (2.3%) with benign MS.

Sample 2 included participants who were recruited into a study of pain as a specific correlate of physical activity and the sample consisted of 28 Caucasian females with an average age of 42.5 (SD = 9.6) years. The participants were primarily employed (n = 22, 78.6%), married (n = 18, 64.3%), and well educated (college graduate n = 20, 71.4%). The average duration since MS diagnosis for Sample 2 was 8.9 (SD = 6.4) years and all participants had relapsing-remitting MS.

Table 1. Participant demographic information for the two independent samples

Variable	Sample 1 (N = 88)		Sample 2 (N = 28)	
	n	%	n	%
Race				
Caucasian	85	96.6	28	100
African American	3	3.4		
Marital Status				
Married	65	73.9	18	64.3
Single	10	11.4	5	17.9
Divorced/separated	10	11.4	3	10.7
Widow/widower	3	3.4	2	7.1
Employment status				
Employed	47	53.4	22	78.6
Unemployed	41	46.6	6	21.4
Education				
High school	20	22.7	2	7.1
Some college	25	28.4	6	21.4
College graduate	43	48.9	20	71.4
Income				
Less than $5,000	1	1.1	1	3.7
$5,001-10,000	0	0	0	0
$10,001-15,000	4	4.5	2	7.4
$15,001-20,000	2	2.3	1	3.7
$20,001-25,000	5	5.7	0	0
$25,001-30,000	4	4.5	0	0
$30,001-40,000	5	5.7	2	7.4

Table 1. (Continued).

Income				
$40,001 or greater	58	65.9	21	77.8
Type of MS				
Variable	Sample 1 (N = 88)		Sample 2 (N = 28)	
	n	%	n	%
Relapsing-remitting	58	65.9	28	100
Secondary progressive	26	29.5	0	0
Primary progressive	1	1.1	0	0
Benign	2	2.3	0	0

Measures

Pain

We measured pain using the short-form of the McGill Pain Questionnaire (SF-MPQ; Melzack, 1987). The SF-MPQ contains a 15-item adjective checklist that assesses sensory (e.g., "stabbing", "sharp") and affective (e.g., "sickening", "tiring-exhausting") dimensions of typical whole body pain intensity. The items are rated using a 4-point intensity scale (0 = none, 1 = mild, 2 = moderate, 3 = severe), and item scores yield sensory (SF-MPQS), affective (SFMPQA), and overall or total (SF-MPQT) pain indices. The SF-MPQ further contains a present pain index (PPI) that assess overall pain intensity using a 6-point scale (0 = none, 1 = mild, 2 = discomforting, 3 = distressing, 4 = horrible, 5 = excruciating). Within the current study, the internal consistency estimates for SF-MPQT, SF-MPQS, and SF-MPQA scores were .90, .88, and .73, respectively, in Sample 1. The internal consistency estimates for SF-MPQT, SF-MPQS, and SF-MPQA scores were .83, .75, and .74, respectively, in Sample 2.

Self-Report Measure of Physical Activity

The Godin Leisure Time Exercise Questionnaire (GLTEQ; Godin and Shephard, 1985) is a self-report measure of physical activity consisting of two questions. The first consists of three open-ended questions asking about the number of times during an average week that vigorous, moderate and mild exercise are undertaken for more than 15 min during free time. Examples of exercise categorized as vigorous included running, swimming, cycling and cross-country skiing activities that were performed at a high intensity. Moderate exercise involved those same types of activities but performed at a lower intensity and other activities such as brisk walking. Mild exercise, which involved minimal effort, included activities such as easy walking, yoga, and golf. The GLTEQ score is calculated by summing the products of the number of times of weekly participation in vigorous, moderate and mild exercise by 9, 5, and 3 METs, respectively. The second question, which asks how often in a typical week exercise that induces sweat is performed, will not be used in the present analyses because of autonomic nervous dysfunction that often affects sweating in individuals with MS. Among individuals with MS, the GLTEQ has been shown to have a moderate to strong correlation with daily accelerometer activity counts ($r = 0.52$, Motl, McAuley, Snook, and Scott, 2006; $r = .53$, Gosney, Scott, Snook, and Motl, 2007).

Objective Measure of Physical Activity

We measured physical activity using the ActiGraph single-axis accelerometer (model 7164 version, Health One Technology, Fort Walton Beach, FL). This accelerometer is a small (2.0 × 1.6 × 0.6 inches) and light weight (1.5 ounces) device that provides an objective, valid, and reliable measure of physical activity for individuals with MS (Gosney et al., 2007; Motl, McAuley, et al., 2006). The Actigraph is powered by a 2430 lithium coin cell battery and contains a single, vertical axis piezoelectric bender element that generates an electrical signal proportional to the force acting on it. Acceleration detection ranges in magnitude from 0.05 - 3.2 Gs and the frequency response ranges from 0.25 - 2.5 Hz. Motion outside normal human movements is rejected by a band-pass filter. The acceleration/deceleration signal is digitized by an analog-to-digital converter and numerically integrated over a pre-programmed epoch interval. At the end of each data collection interval the integrated value of movement counts is stored in RAM and the integrator is reset. The monitor is programmed for start time and data collection interval. The data are retrieved for analysis via a PC interface and software provided with the accelerometers. The movement counts are a summation of positive and negative accelerations measured during a cycle period that is established along with start time during an initialization phase. The counts represent a quantitative measure of activity over time, and are linearly related to the intensity of a participant's physical activity during a cycle period. The epoch in this study was 1 minute. Downloaded data were entered into Microsoft Excel for data processing. The activity counts were summed across each day and the counts from the seven days were then averaged yielding accelerometer data in weekly mean total daily movement counts. The intra-class correlations computed using a two-way model with days as a fixed effect and participants as a random effect for the 7 days of accelerometer data were .91 for Sample 1 and .88 for Sample 2.

Procedure

The procedures for both studies were approved by an institutional review board and all participants in both studies provided written informed consent. Participants in Sample 1 completed a battery of questionnaires assessing MS-related symptoms, including pain, and physical activity, and then wore an accelerometer for 7 consecutive days. Participants received $10 remuneration for completing the study. Participants in Sample 2 completed a battery of questionnaires assessing pain and self-reported physical activity and wore an accelerometer for seven consecutive days. Participants received $25 remuneration for their time.

Data Analysis

Descriptive data are presented as mean ± standard deviation. The relationships between scores from the SF-MPQ, GLTEQ, and accelerometer were analyzed using Pearson product-moment correlations in SPSS, version 15 (SPSS, Chicago, IL). Cohen's (1988) guidelines of .1, .3, and .5 were used for judging the magnitude of the correlations as small, moderate, and large, respectively.

RESULTS

Sample 1

There were 26 individuals with missing accelerometer data, but there were no missing data for the SF-MPQ or GLTEQ. Therefore, mean scores, standard deviations, and correlations involving the accelerometer data are based on a smaller sample of 62 individuals with MS. Mean scores and standard deviations for the SF-MPQ, GLTEQ, and accelerometer are presented in table 2. The mean scores for the physical activity measures from this study were compared with a previous research among 196 individuals with MS (Gosney et al., 2007). The participants in Sample 1 reported lower scores on the GLTEQ (d = –.32) and accumulated fewer accelerometer counts (d = –.26) than the participants of the previous research.

Table 2. Mean scores and standard deviations of study measures in the two independent samples

	Sample 1 (N = 88)			Sample 2 (N = 28)		
Measure	M	SD	Range	M	SD	Range
SF-MPQT	10.7	8.4	0-35	6.1	5.3	0-20
SF-MPQS	7.6	6.4	0-27	4.5	3.8	0-13
SF-MPQA	3.1	2.7	0-10	1.5	1.8	0-7
PPI	1.7	1.0	0-4	1.3	1.2	0-4
GLTEQ	21.6	24.9	0-146	29.1	21.6	0-71
ACCEL	193,524	88,608	41,621-419,893	258,341	131,483	75,978-514,090

Note. SF-MPQT = overall or total score from the adjective checklist portion of the short-form of McGill Pain Questionnaire. SF-MPQS = sensory score from the adjective checklist portion of the short-form of McGill Pain Questionnaire. SF-MPQA = affective score from the adjective checklist portion of the short-form of McGill Pain Questionnaire. PPI = present pain index of the short-form of McGill Pain Questionnaire. GLTEQ = Godin Leisure-Time Exercise Questionnaire. ACCEL = accelerometer.

Table 3 contains the Pearson product-moment correlations among the scores from the SF-MPQ, GLTEQ, and accelerometer. SF-MPQT scores were significantly and inversely correlated with accelerometer activity counts (r = –.29, p = .01), but SF-MPQT scores were not significantly correlated with GLTEQ scores (r = –.08, p = .22). SF-MPQS and SF-MPQA scores were significantly and inversely correlated with accelerometer counts (r = –.22, p = .04; r = –.39, p = .00, respectively), but were not significantly correlated with GLTEQ scores (r = –.07, p = .26; r = –.09, p = .20, respectively). Scatter plots of the significant relationships between accelerometer counts and SF-MPQ scores are provided in figure 1. Similarly, PPI scores were significantly and inversely correlated with accelerometer counts (r = –.29, p = .01), but were not significantly correlated with GLTEQ scores (r = –.03, p = .40). Scores from the GLTEQ were moderate to strongly correlated with accelerometer counts (r = .63, p = .001).

Table 3. Correlations among the measures of pain and physical activity in two independent samples

Measure	Sample 1 (N = 88)				Sample 2 (N = 28)			
	ACCEL		GLTEQ		ACCEL		GLTEQ	
	r	p	r	p	r	p	r	p
SF-MPQT	–.29	.01	–.08	.22	–.40	.02	–.04	.42
SF-MPQS	–.22	.04	–.07	.26	–.40	.02	–.01	.47
SF-MPQA	–.39	.0001	–.09	.20	–.30	.05	–.08	.34
PPI	–.29	.01	–.03	.40	–.45	.01	–.24	.11

Note. SF-MPQT = overall or total score from the adjective checklist portion of the short-form of McGill Pain Questionnaire. SF-MPQS = sensory score from the adjective checklist portion of the short-form of McGill Pain Questionnaire. SF-MPQA = affective score from the adjective checklist portion of the short-form of McGill Pain Questionnaire. PPI = present pain index of the short-form of McGill Pain Questionnaire. GLTEQ = Godin Leisure-Time Exercise Questionnaire. ACCEL = accelerometer.

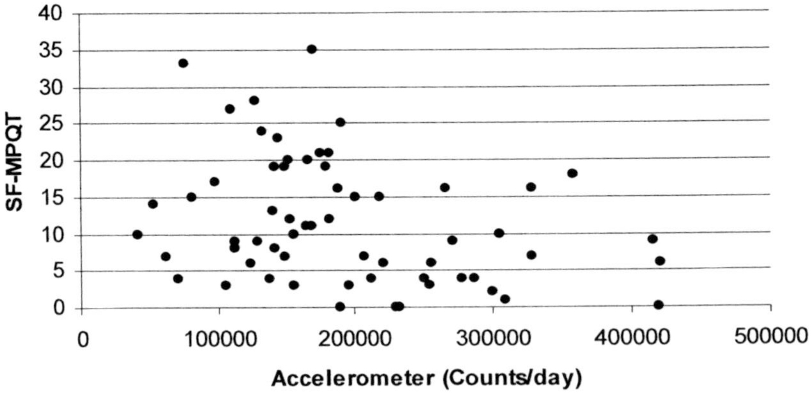

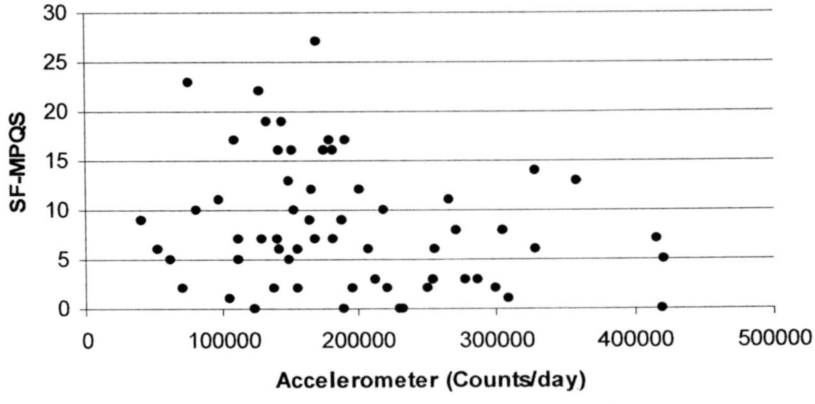

Figure 1. Continued on next page.

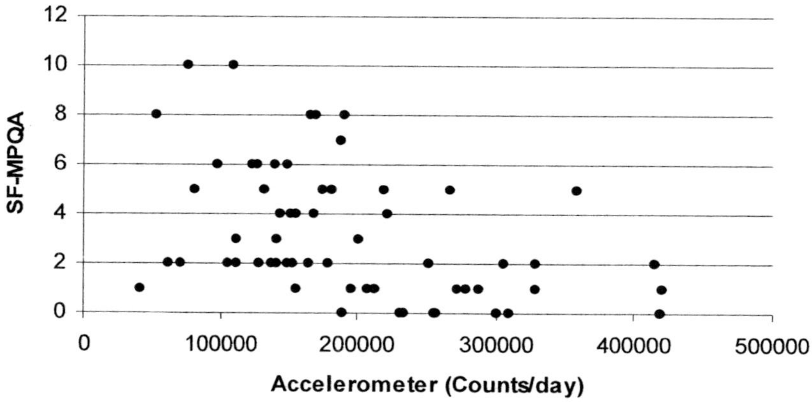

Figure 1. Scatter plots of relationships between accelerometer counts and SF-MPQ overall (SF-MPQT) and sensory (SF-MPQS) and affective (SF-MPQA) subscale scores in Sample 1.

Sample 2

There were 3 individuals with missing accelerometer data, but there were no missing data for the SF-MPQ or GLTEQ. Therefore, mean scores, standard deviations, and correlations involving the accelerometer data are based on a smaller sample of 25 individuals with MS. Mean scores and standard deviations for the measures used in the data analysis are presented in table 2. The mean scores for the physical activity measures from this study were compared with previous research among 196 individuals with MS (Gosney et al., 2007). The participants in Sample 1 reported similar scores on the GLTEQ (d = .00), but accumulated more accelerometer counts (d =.30) than the participants in our previous research.

Table 3 contains the Pearson product-moment correlations among the scores from the SF-MPQ, GLTEQ, and accelerometer. SF-MPQT scores were significantly and inversely correlated with accelerometer activity counts (r = –.40, p = .02), but SF-MPQT scores were not significantly correlated with GLTEQ scores (r = –.04, p = .42). SF-MPQS and SF-MPQA scores were significantly and inversely correlated with accelerometer counts (r = –.40, p = .02; r = –.30, p = .05, respectively), but were not significantly correlated with GLTEQ scores (r = –.01, p = .47; r = –.08, p = .34, respectively). Scatter plots of the significant relationships between accelerometer counts and SF-MPQ scores are provided in figure 2. PPI scores were significantly and inversely correlated with accelerometer counts (r = –.45, p = .01), but PPI scores were not significantly correlated with GLTEQ scores (r = –.24, p = .11). Again, scores from the GLTEQ were moderate to strongly correlated with accelerometer counts (r = .51, p = .005).

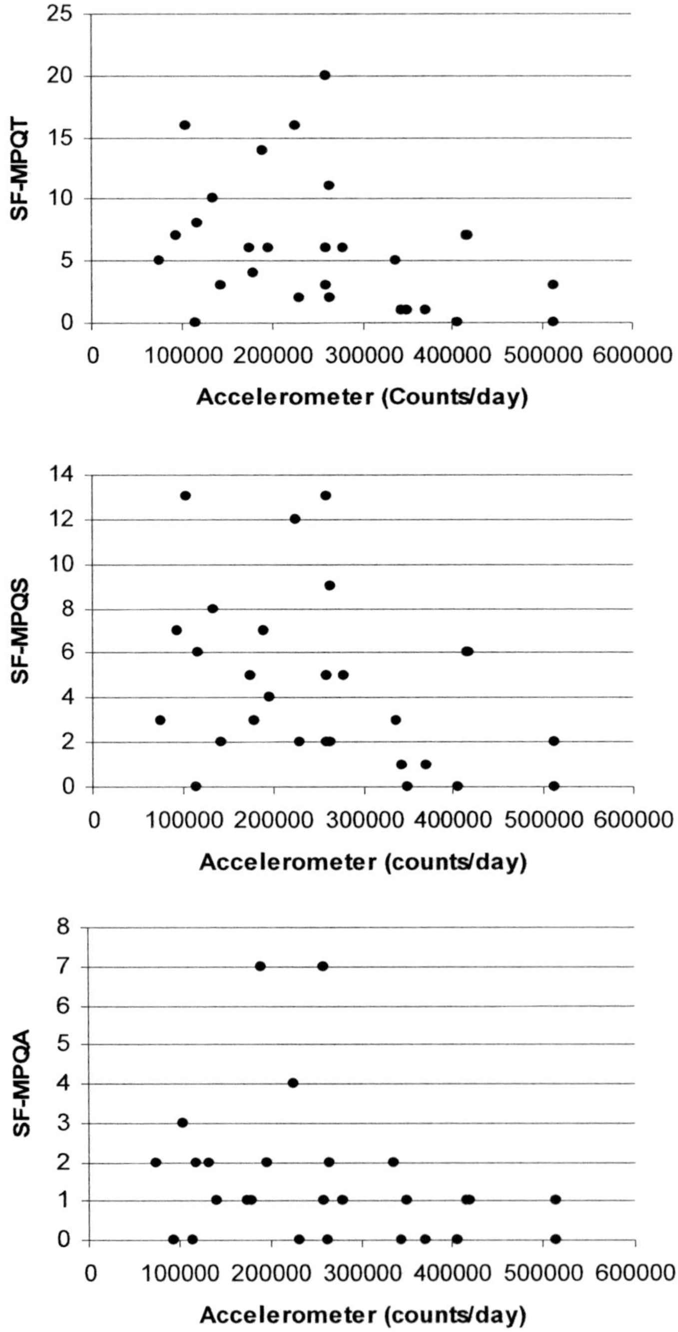

Figure 2. Scatter plots of relationships between accelerometer counts and SF-MPQ overall (SF-MPQT) and sensory (SF-MPQS) and affective (SF-MPQA) subscale scores in Sample 2.

DISCUSSION

This study involved an examination of the relationship between symptoms of pain and physical activity in two samples of individuals with MS. We observed that sensory and affective dimensions of pain as well as the overall intensity of pain were associated with objectively measured physical activity in the two samples of individuals with MS, but there was no evidence that pain was associated with scores on a self-report measure of physical activity. Those who reported greater sensory, affective, and overall pain accumulated fewer activity counts on the accelerometer. The consistent observation of an association between pain and objectively measured physical activity in two samples provides independent support for pain as a possible explanation for the reduction in physical activity among those with MS. Indeed, pain is a common sensory symptom experienced by individuals with MS (Crayton and Rossman, 2006) and is most commonly experienced in the legs as sensations of spasms, aching, and tingling or crawling (Hadjimichael et al., 2007). The pain experienced by those with MS is associated with a variety of functional and behavioral outcomes, including self-reported reductions in mobility and interference with daily activities (Hadjimichael et al., 2007; Svendsen, et al., 2005). The novel finding of this study is that pain is significantly and negatively associated with an objective measure of physical activity in MS.

There was a differential pattern of relationships between pain and physical activity based on the type of physical activity measure. Whereas pain was significantly associated with accelerometer counts, pain was not significantly associated with scores on a self-report measure of physical activity. One potential implication of this differential pattern of relationships is that pain does play a role in physical activity participation, but the relationship is not immediately recognized by participants based on the lack of relationships with the self-report measurement of physical activity. Those who report higher levels of pain intensity are accumulating fewer activity counts as measured by the accelerometer, but are not reporting a reduction in physical activity based on the self-report measure (i.e., GLTEQ). This might suggest that pain-induced reductions in physical activity are inadequately assessed by the GLTEQ, whereas objective measures of physical activity are associated with pain reports. Importantly, the GLTEQ has established evidence that supports the validity of inferences from its scores (Gosney et al., 2007; Motl, McAuley et al., 2006) and scores from the GLTEQ were moderate to strongly correlated with accelerometer counts in both samples included in this study. Therefore, invalid scores on the GLTEQ are likely not an explanation for the lack of an association between pain and physical activity as measured by self-report. Future researchers should consider additional examinations of this differential pattern of relationships between pain and physical activity based on outcome measures and consider possible explanations for the disparate pattern of relationships.

The reason or mechanism for the relationship between pain and physical activity was not examined in this study. One possibility is that movement-induced pain makes the experience of movement unpleasant and so people who experience pain move less. Another possibility is that individuals who experience chronic pain often report fears that movement will exacerbate symptoms (i.e., kinesiophobia; Burwinkle, Robinson, and Turk, 2005). The fear of movement exacerbating pain might result in avoidance of physical activity (Burwinkle et al., 2005). Another possibility is that pain might undermine one's confidence in being physically active. Indeed, pain is moderately and inversely correlated with self-efficacy (e.g., McCahon, Strong,

Sharry, and Cramond, 2005), and perceptions of self-efficacy are considered to be the most powerful predictor of physical activity behavior (McAuley and Blissmer, 2000; Trost, Owen, Bauman, Sallis, and Brown, 2002). Based on a social-cognitive perspective (Bandura, 1986), the experience of pain likely reduces perceptions of self-efficacy and consequently participation in physical activity. Other possibilities include effects of pain on mobility, function, and disability, all of which have been associated with physical activity in individuals with MS (Motl, McAuley et al., 2006; Stuifbergen, Blozis, Harrison, and Becker, 2006). Thus, pain associated with MS may represent a more severe form of the disease that directly impairs physical function and results in reduced physical activity.

The present study has some limitations. One limitation involves the cross-sectional design. This design precludes inferences about the direction of causality among the study variables. For example, participation in physical activity might just as easily affect pain as pain affects physical activity participation. Indeed, social-cognitive theory would support such a position given its foundation in reciprocal determinism (i.e., bi-directional relationships among behavior, the individual, and the environment; Bandura, 1986, 1997). Another limitation is the representativeness of the sample based on the demographic characteristics of the participants and the methods of recruiting participants through self-help groups and MS chapters. Although the descriptive features of our sample are roughly consistent with the demographics of MS (NMSS, 2005), the sample primarily consisted of Caucasian women with relapsing-remitting MS. Future research is warranted that includes more diverse samples consisting of a larger number of men, individuals with primary and secondary progressive MS, and minorities. Despite those limitations, our study provides novel and compelling support for pain as a cross-sectional correlate of objectively measured physical activity among those with MS.

References

Bandura, A. (1986). *Social foundations of thought and action: A social cognitive theory.* Englewood Cliffs, NJ: Prentice Hall.

Bandura, A. (1997). *Self-efficacy: The exercise of control.* New York: John Wiley.

Bouchard, C., and Shephard, R. J. (1994). Physical activity, fitness, and health: The model and key concepts. In C. Bouchard, R. J. Shepard, and T. Stephens (Eds.), *Physical activity, fitness, and health – International proceedings and consensus statement,* (pp. 77 – 88). Human Kinetics: Champaign, IL.

Burwinkle, T., Robinson, J. P., and Turk, D. C. (2005). Fear of movement: Factor structure of the tampa scale of kinesiophobia in patients with fibromyalgia syndrome. The Journal of Pain: *Official Journal of the American Pain Society,* 6(6), 384-391.

Clifford, D. B., and Trotter, J. L. (1984). Pain in multiple sclerosis. *Archives of Neurology,* 41(12), 1270-1272.

Cohen, J. (1988). *Statistical power analysis for the behavioral sciences* (2nd ed.). Hillsdale, NJ: Lawrence Erlbaum Associates.

Crayton, H. J., and Rossman, H. S. (2006). Managing the symptoms of multiple sclerosis: A multimodal approach. *Clinical Therapeutics,* 28(4), 445-460.

Ehde, D. M., Osborne, T. L., Hanley, M. A., Jensen, M. P., and Kraft, G. H. (2006). The scope and nature of pain in persons with multiple sclerosis. *Multiple Sclerosis,* 12(5), 629-638.

Ehde, D. M., Osborne, T. L., and Jensen, M. P. (2005). Chronic pain in persons with multiple sclerosis. *Physical Medicine and Rehabilitation Clinics of North America,* 16(2), 503-512.

Godin, G., and Shephard, R. J. (1985). A simple method to assess exercise behavior in the community. *Canadian Journal of Applied Sport Sciences,* 10(3), 141-146.

Gosney, J. L., Scott, J. A., Snook, E. M., and Motl, R. W. (2007). Physical activity and multiple sclerosis: Validity of self-report and objective measures. *Family and Community Health,* 30, 144-150.

Hadjimichael, O., Kerns, R. D., Rizzo, M. A., Cutter, G., and Vollmer, T. (2007). Persistent pain and uncomfortable sensations in persons with multiple sclerosis. *Pain,* 127(1-2), 35-41.

International Association for the Study of Pain. (1979). Pain terms: A list with definitions and notes on usage. *Pain,* 6, 249.

Kalia, L. V., and O'Connor, P. W. (2005). Severity of chronic pain and its relationship to quality of life in multiple sclerosis. *Multiple Sclerosis,* 11(3), 322 – 327.

Lublin, F. D. (2005). Clinical features and diagnosis of multiple sclerosis. *Neurologic Clinics,* 23, 1-15.

McAuley, E., and Blissmer, B. (2000). Self-efficacy determinants and consequences of physical activity. *Exercise and Sport Sciences Reviews,* 28(2), 85-88.

McCahon, S., Strong, J., Sharry, R., and Cramond, T. (2005). Self-report and pain behavior among patients with chronic pain. *The Clinical Journal of Pain,* 21(3), 223-231.

Melzack, R. (1987). The short-form McGill pain questionnaire. *Pain,* 30(2), 191-197.

Motl, R. W., Arnett, P. A., Smith, M. M., Barwick, F. H., Ahlstrom, B., and Stover, E. J. (in press). Worsening of symptoms is associated with lower physical activity levels in individuals with multiple sclerosis. *Multiple Sclerosis.*

Motl, R. W., McAuley, E., and Snook, E. M. (2005). Physical activity and multiple sclerosis: A meta-analysis. *Multiple Sclerosis,* 11(4), 459-463.

Motl, R. W., McAuley, E., Snook, E. M., and Scott, J. A. (2006). Validity of physical activity measures in ambulatory individuals with multiple sclerosis. *Disability and Rehabilitation,* 28(18), 1151-1156.

Motl, R. W., Snook, E. M., McAuley, E., and Gliottoni, R. C. (2006). Symptoms, self-efficacy, and physical activity among individuals with multiple sclerosis. *Research in Nursing and Health,* 29(6), 597-606.

National Multiple Sclerosis Society. (2005). *Multiple sclerosis information sourcebook.* New York, NY: Information Resource Center and Library of the National Multiple Sclerosis Society.

Schapiro, R. T. (2003). *Managing the symptoms of multiple sclerosis.* (4th ed.). New York: Demos Medical Publishing.

Solaro, C., Brichetto, G., Amato, M. P., Cocco, E., Colombo, B., D'Aleo, G., et al. (2004). The prevalence of pain in multiple sclerosis: A multicenter cross-sectional study. *Neurology,* 63(5), 919-921.

Solaro, C., Lunardi, G. L., and Mancardi, G. L. (2003). Pain and MS. *International MS Journal/MS Forum,* 10(1), 14-19.

Stenager, E., Knudsen, L., and Jensen, K. (1991). Acute and chronic pain syndromes in multiple sclerosis. *Acta Neurologica Scandinavica,* 84(3), 197-200.

Stenager, E., Knudsen, L., and Jensen, K. (1995). Acute and chronic pain syndromes in multiple sclerosis. A 5-year follow-up study. *Italian Journal of Neurological Sciences,* 16(9), 629-632.

Stuifbergen, A. K., Blozis, S. A., Harrison, T. C., and Becker, H. A. (2006). Exercise, functional limitations, and quality of life: A longitudinal study of persons with multiple sclerosis. *Archives of Physical Medicine and Rehabilitation,* 87(7), 935-943.

Svendsen, K. B., Jensen, T. S., Hansen, H. J., and Bach, F. W. (2005). Sensory function and quality of life in patients with multiple sclerosis and pain. *Pain,* 114(3), 473-481.

Svendsen, K. B., Jensen, T. S., Overvad, K., Hansen, H. J., Koch-Henriksen, N., and Bach, F. W. (2003). Pain in patients with multiple sclerosis: A population-based study. *Archives of Neurology,* 60(8), 1089-1094.

Trost, S. G., Owen, N., Bauman, A. E., Sallis, J. F., and Brown, W. (2002). Correlates of adults' participation in physical activity: Review and update. *Medicine and Science in Sports and Exercise,* 34(12), 1996-2001.

In: Exercise and Women's Health
Editor: Laura A. Charlington, pp. 113-126
ISBN: 978-1-60456-013-8

Chapter 5

PERCEIVED, DESIRED, AND ACTUAL BODY IMAGE: A COMPARISON OF HUMAN KINETICS AND NON HUMAN KINETICS STUDENTS

Kara L. Latter and Angela M. Thompson*
Department of Human Kinetics, St. Francis Xavier University

ABSTRACT

This chapter provides the results of a study that compared the perceived, desired, and actual body images of 20 female students at a relatively small, primarily undergraduate university. Ten females were enrolled in a Human Kinetics (HK) program while the other 10 females were enrolled in other programs (Non-HK). Perceived and desired body images were determined from self-reported responses to a body image questionnaire. This body image questionnaire featured two questions associated with nine silhouettes that ranged in size from emaciated to obese. Actual body image was determined from anthropometric measurements and the applicable calculations for somatotype using the Heath-Carter Somatotype Calculations procedures. Descriptive statistics including means ± standard deviation were calculated for each group (i.e., HK and Non-HK) and the groups' perceived, desired, and actual body images compared using Oneway Analyses of Variance (ANOVA). Although, there were no significant differences ($p = .105$) in the body image satisfaction/dissatisfaction experienced between the HK and Non-HK groups, a high percentage (i.e., 70%) of the female students desired a smaller body image than what she perceived for herself. The ability to accurately identify one's actual body image was also not significantly ($p = .151$) different between the two groups. In fact, few females (i.e., 20%) accurately identified their body image from the nine silhouettes presented on the questionnaire. Thus, it was concluded that even though the female HK students were expected to know more about their body, including how and why their body moves, as well as a greater level of comfort with their physical body and how it moves, no significant differences existed in the perceived, desired, and actual body

* Corresponding Author: Angela M. Thompson, Ph.D.; Department of Human Kinetics, St. Francis Xavier University, P.O. Box 5000, 1 West Street; Antigonish, NS, CANADA; B2G 2W5; Phone: 902-867-3540; Fax: 902-867-3904; Email: amthomps@stfx.ca

images of these female students compared to other females enrolled in Non-HK programs at a relatively small, primarily undergraduate university.

INTRODUCTION

One would expect college or university students enrolled in a physical education-type program such as Human Kinetics, Human Movement Studies, or Kinesiology to be more aware of the positive health-related benefits of physical activity compared to students enrolled in various other programs. It is also realistic to assume that those students enrolled in these types of programs would have a better understanding of how and why their bodies move and as a result be able to move their bodies more effectively and experience more satisfaction or physical self-esteem as a result. It is also believed that these students are more likely to be more physically fit than students enrolled in other programs simply because of a greater participation in physical activities such as exercise and training. It is questionable however, as to whether or not this higher level of knowledge, comfort with one's physical body, and a higher level of physical fitness is associated with a better, more accurate - or healthier - perception of one's body image or less of a desire to change one's body image.

Body image is defined as "a subjective picture of one's own physical appearance established by self-observation and by noting the reactions of others" (Merriam-Webster, 2002). Body image dissatisfaction then refers to an unhappiness or displeasure with one's physical or outward appearance. When an individual's perceived and desired body images do not match, he or she is said to be dissatisfied with his or her body image. Generally, body image dissatisfaction increases with age in girls, with one study reporting that 76% of post-pubertal girls desired a smaller physique than the one they perceived they had (Thompson and Chad, 2000). Given the increase in body dissatisfaction with age, it is no surprise that the college or university years are a time in which many students experience some level of body image dissatisfaction with most studies indicating greater dissatisfaction amongst females (Stuhldreher and Ryan, 1999). Although this trend has been evident for many years, the gap between male and female body image dissatisfaction has not increased or decreased over time. (Rozin, Trachtenberg, and Cohen, 2001).

There are a number of factors proposed to relate to the experience of body image satisfaction/dissatisfaction in females. One such factor is the print media. In one study, females were left waiting in a room with either newspapers or fashion magazines (Turner, Hamilton, Jacobs, Angood, and Dwyer, 1997). These females were then asked to complete a three-part questionnaire that included choosing the silhouette that best represented their body shape as well as a series of questions relating to their perceptions of their bodies and dieting behaviors. The females who looked at the fashion magazines were found to be less satisfied with their body image compared to the females who only had newspapers to look at while waiting. This suggests that the media - and the images presented within - play a role in body image dissatisfaction in females.

It is also possible that one's area of study influences their body image satisfaction/dissatisfaction. As previously noted, one would expect female students who learn about the human body and specifically how and why it moves and how to move it effectively and efficiently, are more likely to be able to move it well and as a result have higher levels of physical self-esteem than other females. These females, one would assume would experience less body dissatisfaction than other females who are less "in tune" with their bodies. Further, one might assume that more physically fit females would also experience less body dissatisfaction than their less fit counterparts. Physical fitness may also relate to program of study in that one would expect Human Kinetics (along with similar programs of study) students to be more physically fit simply to "practice what they preach" or to "practice what they learn".

Many studies have examined body image, particularly in females. Of these studies, most researchers used some sort of body image questionnaire or scale (i.e. two-dimensional silhouettes) to obtain an indication of a female's body image and in turn from her responses determine her body image satisfaction/dissatisfaction. Specifically, females are asked to select an image from the series of silhouettes presented on the questionnaire that they think best represents the outward physical appearance of their body. They are also asked which of the silhouettes presented they would desire for themselves. It is in comparing these two responses that body image satisfaction/dissatisfaction is determined. Thus these series of two-dimensional silhouettes that represent the outward shape or appearance of the body have been used to assess body image in different populations including females of all ages, many ethnicities, as well as in females with eating disorders (DiGioacchine, Sargent, and Topping, 2001; Leonhard and Barry, 1998; Manley, Tonkin, and Hammons, 1988; Shih and Kubo, 2004; Tehard, Van Liere, Com Nougué, and Clavel-Chapelon, 2002; Turner et al., 1997). Two reasons for the frequent use of this type of assessment are because it is cost-effective and easy to administer since it does not require the research participant to recall numerical values such as body weight or body fat percentage when choosing their perceived and desired body images. Although some researchers think that the silhouettes give an "unrealistic representation of the human form" (Thompson and Gray, 1995), the majority of researchers prefer to use them over other methods when comparing body image among two or more groups of subjects. Whether researchers used silhouettes from past research or created their own set, it appears that this method of self report is a popular choice for determining body image satisfaction/dissatisfaction and has proven to be a relatively valid and reliable measure (Tehard, et al., 2002).

Although there are other series of silhouettes available (Carroll, Gleeson, Ribsby, and Dugdale, 1986; Dwyer, Feldman, Seltser, and Mayer, 1969), the series of silhouettes created by Stunkard, Sorenson, and Schulsinger (1983) appear frequently in the literature. Stunkard et al. (1983) created nine silhouettes for females (there is also a series of nine silhouettes for males) ranging from emaciated to obese (see Figure 1). Using these silhouettes, subjects are asked to respond to two questions related to their body image. These questions typically ask (1) which of the silhouettes most looks like your body? and (2) which of the silhouettes would you desire for yourself? Using the responses to these two questions, body image satisfaction/dissatisfaction can be determined. Specifically, if the silhouettes chosen in response to both questions are the same, the subject is classified as *satisfied* with her body shape (i.e., her perceived and desired body shapes are the same). However, if the perceived body shape is smaller or larger than the desired body shape, the subject is then classified with a *dissatisfied* body image. It should be pointed out that in most studies of females' body image; few subjects desire a larger body shape than what they currently perceive themselves to have (Thompson and Chad, 2005).

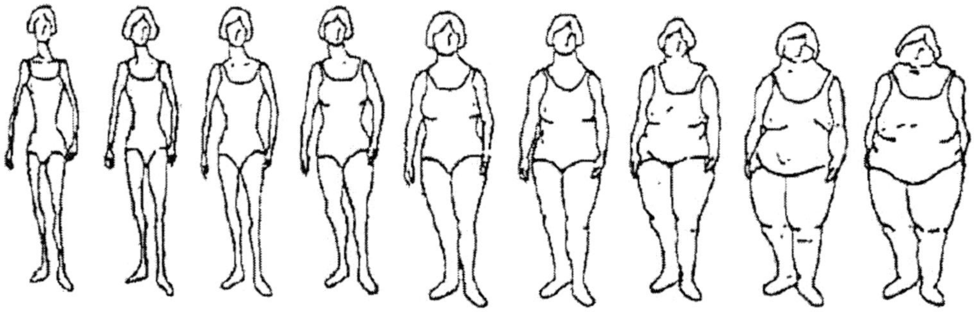

Figure 1. Nine female silhouettes ranging from emaciated to obese (Stunkard et al.,1983).

Although the series of silhouettes are useful for determining *perceived* and *desired* body images, they do not indicate *actual* body image. If an individual has a *distorted* body image or perceptual deficits, he or she may not be able to correctly perceive his or her body image when looking at a series of silhouettes. In this instance, he or she is likely to choose a silhouette that is larger or smaller than his or her actual shape. This was noted in a study of body image in young females with and without eating disorders. Specifically, Manley et al. (1988) conducted a study in which females with anorexia nervosa or bulimia nervosa as well as a control group of females without an eating disorder were presented eleven different cards with a profile and frontal pictures of various female figures. These females were then asked which profile they felt best represented (1) the way they saw themselves in the mirror, (2) the way they thought they looked (i.e., without a mirror image), (3) the way they felt they looked (i.e., how they physically felt), and (4) the way they wanted to look. The findings from this study indicated that the females with eating disorders idealized (i.e., desired) a thinner shape than females without an eating disorder. Further, the females with an eating disorder overestimated their actual body shape to a greater extent. In other words, these females were not able to accurately identify their own body shape from the series of silhouettes on the questionnaire.

One's actual body image or outward appearance (i.e., somatotype) can be determined from frontal, side and rear-view photographs and classified according to an established series of photographs developed by Sheldon and colleagues (Sheldon, Dupertuis, and McDermott, 1954; Sheldon, Stevens, and Tucker, 1940) or anthropometrically measured and calculated using the Heath-Carter Somatotype Calculation forms. Both classification procedures results in the determination of one's somatotype. Somatotype is the term used to describe the outward appearance or physique of the body and consists of three relatively independent, but highly related components: endomorphy, mesomorphy and ectomorphy (Malina, Bouchard, and Bar-Or, 2004). Endomorphy refers to the relative fatness of the body. More specifically, endomorphy refers to the softness and roundness of the body as well as the predominance of the digestive organs. Mesomorphy, or relative muscularity, is characterized by the definition of the muscles, bones and connective tissue. Ectomorphy refers to the relative linearity of the body and refers to a high body surface area to body mass ratio.

To supplement the adult resources for classifying individual somatotypes created by Sheldon and colleagues (Sheldon et al., 1940; Sheldon et al., 1954), Tanner and Whitehouse (1982) created the *Atlas of Children's Growth: Normal Variation and Growth Disorders* which illustrates the growth patterns of various somatotypes in boys and girls who are healthy and in those who have growth disorders. A total of twenty girls were photographed from age six to full maturity (i.e., 16 to 19 years of age) allowing for a complete visual of each somatotype in the development process and when fully mature. These photographs are useful for comparing the shape - or somatotype - of silhouettes used to determine body image in developing and developed females.

Primarily because of ethical concerns, front, side and back view photographs of physiques are seldom taken to determine individual somatotype. Rather, the three somatotype components are calculated using the Heath-Carter Somatotype Calculation procedures along with the following anthropometric measurements: stretched stature, body mass, triceps, subscapular, suprailliac, and calf skinfolds, flexed arm and calf girths, and humerus and femur breadths. The result is a three number rating (i.e., 4-5-3) or description of one's somatotype listed in the order of endomorphy-mesomorphy-ectomorphy. A lower number indicates a lower amount of the specified characteristic. For example, an individual high in endomorphy (i.e., relative fatness), average in mesomorphy (i.e., relative muscularity) and low in endomorphy (i.e., relative linearity) could have the following somatotype: 5-3-1 and be classified as a meso-endomorph. The average female somatotype is 4.5-3.5-2.5, a meso-endomorph (Malina et al, 2004). This average female somatotype can be described as predominantly rounder and softer, with moderate muscle definition, and a lower body surface area to mass ratio.

Sobral and Vasconcelos (1996) conducted a study in which somatotype photographs were converted into silhouettes. Females in secondary school were first measured for somatotype and then asked to choose their perceived body image, desired body image, and the image they found most appealing amongst the silhouettes presented. The results from this study showed that these females tended to have actual physiques or somatotypes that were highest in endomorphy, yet preferred somatotypes that were more ectomorphic. In other words, these females preferred a body image less round, less soft, and more linear or thinner than what they actually had.

Since somatotype is based on the concept of the relationship between three components of the body, relating to the individual's physique, one might assume that the somatotype is the objective concept of one's physical appearance (Malina et al, 2004), while body image refers to the subjective concept of one's physical appearance (Merriam-Webster, 2002). The relationship between body image and somatotype has not been fully explored. Furthermore, the relationship of these two variables has not been compared in individuals who have a greater interest and knowledge of Human Kinetics compared to those without this interest and not enrolled in this sort of program of study.

Given that the objective and subjective views of the body have not been fully explored (i.e., the relationship between body image and somatotype) and in particular in students enrolled in a program of study that emphasizes a greater understanding of human movement, the purpose of the study reported in this chapter was to compare the perceived, desired, and actual body shapes of Human Kinetics versus non Human Kinetics female students. It was hypothesized that a greater percentage of the females enrolled in the Human Kinetics program would perceive their body image more accurately than the females enrolled in other programs. It was further hypothesized that the Human Kinetics group would report less body image dissatisfaction than the female students in the Non-Human Kinetics programs, that is, a smaller percentage of students from Human Kinetics programs would prefer a smaller physique to what they perceived they had.

METHODS

Subjects

Through an email invitation, more than 100 females in their fourth year of study from a relatively small, primarily undergraduate university were invited to participate in this study. Twenty females agreed to participate (representing a 20% response rate); half of the subjects (i.e., 10) were enrolled in the Human Kinetics program while the remaining half (i.e., 10) were enrolled in other programs. Ethical approval for this study was obtained from the local university's Research Ethics Board and informed consent obtained from each subject prior to data collection.

Procedures

This study included two distinct components – determination of *perceived* and *desired* body shape to determine body image satisfaction/dissatisfaction and the measurement of somatotype to determine actual body image.

Body Image Questionnaire

To determine perceived and desired body image, each female participant was asked two questions in relation to the series of nine silhouettes created by Stunkard et al. (1983):

A. Which figure do you feel best represents your actual body image?
B. Which figure would you most like to look like?

Each female was asked to place the letters "A" and "B" corresponding to her answers under the applicable silhouette.

The nine silhouettes ranged from extremely thin or emaciated to extremely fat or obese. These silhouettes were presented to each female on an 8.5" x 11" (216 x 279 mm) sheet of paper resulting in a silhouette height of approximately six centimeters. As previously noted, these silhouettes have been found to be effective for determining body image because there are no numbers associated with them and it is simply a case of deciding which silhouette best represents one's body and which silhouette one most desires or prefers to have (Leonard and Barry, 1998; Rozin et al, 2001; Stuhldreher and Ryan, 1999; Tehard et al, 2002; Turner et al, 1997). Although previous studies have also shown that more accurate assessments of body image are found when the silhouettes are life size (Holder and Keates, 2006), creating this type of scale was not feasible for this study.

Somatotype

Actual body image was determined for each female using the silhouettes and her individually measured and calculated somatotype. In doing so, according to the protocols identified by the International Society for the Advancement in Kinanthropometry (ISAK, 2001), the following anthropometric measurements were taken by a Certified Fitness Consultant (CFC)-trained researcher (Canadian Physical Activity, Fitness and Lifestyle

Approach, 2004): stretched stature, body mass, triceps, subscapular, suprailliac, and calf skinfolds, femur and humerus breadths, and flexed arm and flexed calf girths. Stretched stature was measured from each female in socked feet using a wall stadiometer to the nearest 0.1 cm. Body mass was also taken in socked feet with shorts and a tank top (or small t-shirt) and measured on a calibrated electronic scale to the nearest 0.1 kg. The four skinfold measurements (triceps, subscapular, suprailliac, and calf), were taken using Harpenden skinfold calipers from the right hand side of the body and recorded to the nearest 0.1 mm. The two width measurements (humerus and femur) and two girth measurements (flexed arm and calf) were taken using bone calipers and a measuring tape respectively. All anthropometric measurements were taken by the CFC-trained researcher in a private setting to ensure the subject's comfort. Two measurements were taken at each measurement site and then averaged. If the first two measurements differed by more than 0.4 mm for stretched stature, 0.4 kg for body mass, 0.4 mm for skinfolds, 0.4 mm for breadths, or 0.4 mm for girths, a third measurement was taken and the median value recorded.

Data Analysis

Body Image Satisfaction/Dissatisfaction (Perceived – Desired)

The silhouette that each female chose as what she considered to most closely resemble her body image was called her "perceived body image". The silhouette identified as the body image she preferred was called her "desired body image". When these two silhouettes differed (i.e., perceived and desired), she was classified as having a dissatisfied body image, if they differed by two or more silhouettes, she was classified as "very dissatisfied" with her body image. When the two chosen silhouettes were the same, the female was classified as "satisfied" with her body shape.

Body Image Misperception (Somatotype – Perceived)

Actual body shape was determined from the silhouettes and the individually calculated somatotype. Somatotypes were calculated using the following formulas for the specific somatotype components (i.e., endomorphy, mesomorphy, ectomorphy) obtained from the Heath-Carter Somatotype Calculation procedures:

These calculations resulted in a numeric value or rating for endomorphy, mesomorphy, and ectomorphy for each female and were then compared to the previously established somatotype ratings given to each silhouette from figure 1. Models from the *Atlas of Children's Growth: Normal Variation and Growth Disorders* (Tanner and Whitehouse, 1982) were used to provide a somatotype rating for each of the nine silhouettes used in this study. Although each component of the somatotype was considered, a greater emphasis was placed on the endomorphic component. As such, the first silhouette had an endomorphic rating of '1", the second silhouette, an endomorphic rating of "2" and so forth. Figure 2 provides an illustrative comparison of the fourth silhouette and its matching somatotype.

Thus in this study, the actual body shape of each female was the silhouette with the same endomorphic component as calculated for her individually determined somatotype. Using this method, females whose *perceived* and *actual* body shapes did not match were considered to have an incorrect perception of their body image while those whose *perceived* and *actual* body shapes did match were classified as having a correct perception. Thus, for data analysis and presentation, females whose perceived body image matched their actual body image were placed in the "correct perception" category while those who had a different perception of their actual body image were placed in either the "larger incorrect perception" category (i.e., believed her body to be larger than what it actually was) or the "smaller incorrect perception" category (i.e., believed her body to be smaller than it actually was).

$$\text{Endomorphy} = -0.7182 + 0.1451(X) - 0.00068(X^2) + 0.0000014(X^3)$$

where X = the sum of triceps, subscapular and suprailliac skinfolds in mm.

Mesomorphy = 0.858 (humerus breadth in cm) + 0.601 (femur breadth in cm) + 0.188 (corrected arm girth in cm) + 0.161 (corrected calf girth in cm) – 0.131 (height in cm) + 4.5

where corrected arm girth = flexed arm girth (cm) minus the triceps skinfold (cm)

where corrected calf girth = calf girth (cm) minus the medial calf skinfold (cm).

If HWR > 40.74, Ectomorphy = 0.732 (HWR) – 28.58

If $39.65 < \text{HWR} \leq 40.74$, Ectomorphy = 0.463 (HWR) – 17.615

If HWR ≤ 39.65), Ectomorphy= 0.5

where Height-Weight Ratio (HWR) is height (cm) divided by the cube root of weight (kg).

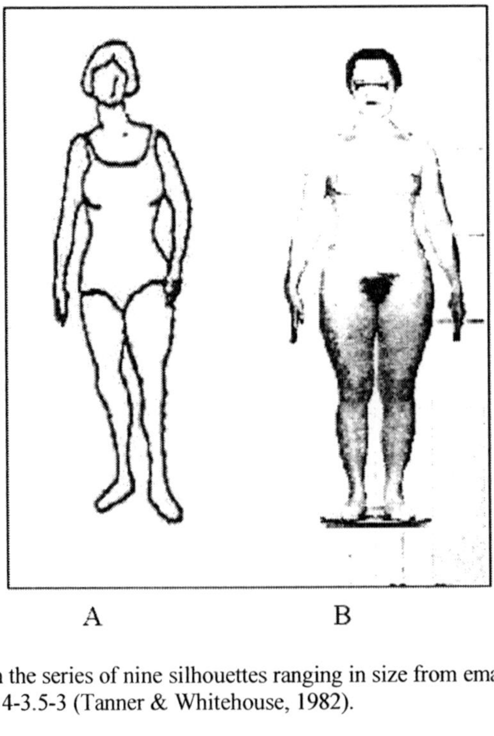

A B

Figure 2. A The fourth from the series of nine silhouettes ranging in size from emaciated to obese (Stunkard et al., 1983). B Somatotype 4-3.5-3 (Tanner & Whitehouse, 1982).

Descriptive statistics (mean ± standard deviation) were calculated for the total sample and for each group (HK; Non-HK) for age, height, weight, sum of skinfolds, and the somatotype components endomorphy, mesomorphy, and ectomorphy. The mode or most frequently reported silhouette was also determined for perceived, desired, and actual body image for each group of students. One-way analyses of variance (ANOVA) were used to compare the two groups for perceived, desired, and actual body images. A p value of less than .05 was chosen to denote significance.

RESULTS

Twenty females volunteered to participate in this study. Ten of these females were enrolled in the Human Kinetics program while the other ten were enrolled in Psychology, Sociology, Biology, Human Nutrition, Nursing, and English. Descriptive statistics of the anthropometric variables for the Human Kinetics (HK) and Non-Human Kinetics (Non-HK) groups are presented in Table 1. Although the Non-HK females were slightly heavier, had a greater sum of four skinfolds, and higher endomorphy values than the HK females, these differences were not significant.

Table 1. Anthropometric variables (mean ± standard deviation) for the HK* and Non-HK females students, and for the total sample

	HK Students (n = 10)	Non-HK Students (n = 10)	Total Sample (n = 20)
Age	21.2 ± 0.8	21.4 ± 0.7	21.3 ± 0.7
Height (cm)	166.2 ± 5.9	165.0 ± 9.0	165.6 ± 7.4
Weight (kg)	61.6 ± 6.9	62.3 ± 10.5	165.6 ± 8.7
Sum Skinfolds (mm)	44.5 ± 8.2	50.4 ± 11.9	47.4 ± 10.4
Endomorphy	4.4 ± 0.7	4.9 ± 1.0	4.7 ± 0.9
Mesomorphy	3.9 ± 0.8	4.1 ± 1.5	4.0 ±1.2
Ectomorphy	2.3 ± 0.7	2.2 ± 1.4	2.2 ± 1.1

* HK = Human Kinetics.

The data presented in table 2 shows the modes of the perceived, desired, and actual body image choices for the HK and Non-HK groups. There were no significant differences in perceived, desired, or actual body images between the HK and Non-HK groups of females. Out of the ten HK students, only two were satisfied with their perceived body image, six were dissatisfied, and two were very dissatisfied (i.e., preferred a silhouette two or more smaller than their perceived silhouette). For the ten Non-HK students, four were satisfied, five dissatisfied, and one very dissatisfied with their body image. It is important to point out that no female preferred a silhouette bigger than what she perceived for herself. Thus, all females in this study dissatisfied with their body image preferred a smaller shape.

Table 2. Most frequent silhouette choice of HK* and Non-HK female students for body image

Body Image	HK Students	Non-HK Students	p value
Perceived BI**	4	4	.722
Desired BI***	3	3	.105
Actual BI****	4	5	.151

* HK = Human Kinetics

** Perceived BI (Body Image) refers to the silhouette chosen as the body image which best represented what the subjects perceived they looked like.

*** Desired BI (Body Image) refers to the silhouette chosen as the body image which the subjects would most prefer to look like.

**** Actual BI (Body Image) refers to the individual's actual body image as determined from individually measured and calculated somatotypes.

The HK students had an average somatotype of 4.5-4.0-2.4 while the Non-HK students' average somatotype was 5.0-4.1-2.2. Although the average somatotype is referred to as a meso-endomorph for both groups, it should be noted that the Non-HK students had higher values of endomorphy. This indicates that the Non-HK females had, on average, higher levels of relative fatness. The mode endomorphic component for each group correlated directly with the actual body image for both groups at silhouette number 4. Figure 3 shows a somatoplot (i.e., two-dimensional graph of somatotypes) of the somatotypes of each female that participated in this study as well as the average value for the HK and Non-HK groups. It can be seen from the somatoplot that there was greater variability in the somatotypes of the Non-HK females with a range of 3.6-1.5-4.4 to 6.5-6.0-0.5 noted.

Four of the HK students had a correct perception of their body image (i.e., perceived and actual body images matched). Of the six HK females with an incorrect perception of her body image, three perceived their body as larger than it actually was and the other three smaller. Similarly, four of the Non-HK students had correct perceptions of their body shape while one female incorrectly perceived her body shape to be larger than it actually was while the other five females perceived their body shape to be smaller than reality.

Discussion

The purpose of this study was to compare the perceived, desired, and actual body images of Human Kinetics (HK) and Non Human Kinetics (Non-HK) females at a relatively small, primarily undergraduate university. It was hypothesized that the HK students would be better able to predict their actual body shape and that they would be less likely to desire a smaller body image than the students in the Non-HK group. Twenty female students provided data for this study with perceived and desired body image determined from a self-report body image questionnaire and actual body image determined from anthropometric measurements and calculations to determine somatotype.

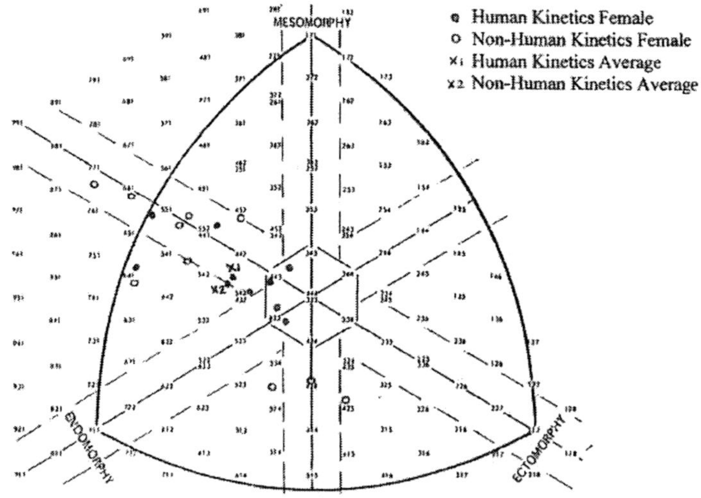

Figure 3. Somatoplot of Human Kinetics and Non-Human Kinetics students' somatotypes.

The results of the study indicated no significant differences between the two groups of students. In other words, HK students were not any better at identifying their actual body image compared to the Non-HK students, rejecting the first hypothesis. The second hypothesis was also rejected in that the females in the HK group were no more satisfied with their current body image, or desiring less of a change in body image compared to the Non-HK students. Although there were no significant differences amongst these two groups, overall most females in this study did experience some dissatisfaction with their body image in that they desired a body shape smaller than what they perceived they had. This is consistent with previous research conducted on females in this age group (Stuhldreher and Ryan, 1999). Further most females in this study had difficulties in correctly identifying their actual body image.

One major difference found in this study compared to previous research was how the females incorrectly identified their body image in that most under-estimated their actual body image. Previous studies indicated that most females chose a silhouette more endomorphic than what they actually were, indicating that they perceived themselves to be larger than their actual body size (Sobral and Vasconcelos, 1996). In this study, however, 66% (i.e., 8/12 females who incorrectly identified their actual shape) estimated their body size as smaller than it actually was, indicating that body image misperception or distortion can go both ways and that some females may actually think they are smaller than what they really are. It is important to note however that in making comparisons to past research, that different methodologies were used - in particular for determining actual body image. Frequently in past research, actual body shape was determined solely by the researcher looking at their subject and choosing which silhouette they felt best represented his or her body shape (Holder and Keates, 2006; Manley et al., 1988). It is possible that determining actual body image with somatotypes (endomorphy, mesomorphy, ectomorphy) results in a much different estimation of body image than an overall visual appraisal. Although a visual appraisal may work when estimating obesity as was noted by Mueller, Joos, and Schull (1985) in their validation of the use of silhouettes for classifying females as normal weight, overweight and obese in skilled observers. In addition to calculating somatotypes from anthropometric measurements, greater emphasis was placed on the endomorphy component of somatotype in this study where as

Sobral and Vasconcelos (1996) used somatotype photographs modified into silhouettes, which considered all three components of the somatotype.

It is important to point out that 70% of the females in this study – regardless of program of study were either dissatisfied or very dissatisfied with their current body image. This value is similar to the body image dissatisfaction found in previous studies (Holder and Keates, 2006; Manley et al., 1998; Sobral and Vasconcelos, 1996). Furthermore, it should be pointed out that all females, both in this study and in the previously mentioned research, who experienced some sort of dissatisfaction with their body image, preferred a body image that was one to two silhouettes smaller than what they perceived their body image to be (Holder and Keates, 2006; Manley et al., 1998; Sobral and Vasconcelos, 1996).

One strength of this study was that an objective measurement was made of each females' actual body image. Another related strength was that all anthropometric measurements were taken by the same CFC-trained researcher. Limitations to this study include the small sample size, the lack of ethnic variation in the sample, and the reality of the silhouettes used in the body image questionnaire. Specifically, the shape of some of the silhouettes may result in some participants finding it difficult to find themselves in one of them. The legs, especially in the thinner figures seemed disproportionate to the rest of the body, and the variance between each figure often times was not equal. One final limitation of the study relates to participant recruitment. It is likely that those who volunteered to participate felt more comfortable with their body image as testing required anthropometric measurements such as weight and skinfolds. Persons who are more comfortable in having these measurements taken were probably less likely to have major body image dissatisfactions or severely inaccurate perceptions of their actual body image. This was shown in the results as more subjects predicted a smaller silhouette for their perceived body image when in fact they were larger. Also, the simple fact that these persons were more confident in their body shape (i.e., had a higher level of physical self esteem) would also be a reason for participating whereas the people who suffered from severe body image dissatisfaction would not consider volunteering for such a study.

CONCLUSION

In conclusion, it was found that there was no significant difference in the perceived, desired, and actual body images when comparing Human Kinetics to Non- Human Kinetics female students. Thus, these results should be considered when one assumes that because Human Kinetics students are likely more knowledgeable about their bodies, that does not mean they can better predict their actual body image. Also, one should not assume that the physical fitness levels usually associated with being a Human Kinetics student do not indicate - or relate to - a greater satisfaction with their current body image. Future research should be conducted to further examine the qualitative aspects of the study such as why female students are dissatisfied with their current body image, and what it is that causes them to incorrectly identify their body image. One could also determine if there are different reasons for the perceived and desired body images amongst the two groups of students (HK vs. Non-HK). Furthermore, future research should examine body dissatisfaction as a whole amongst females and ways in which we can try to reduce the number of people who are dissatisfied as well as the amount of dissatisfaction experienced. Finally, more research should be conducted to create a more realistic, life-like scale of body silhouettes for subjects to choose from for future research on body image.

REFERENCES

Bartsch, A. J., Brümmerhoff, A., Greil, H., and Neumärker, K. (2003). Shall the anthropometry of physique cast new light on the diagnoses and treatment of eating disorders? *European Child and Adolescent Psychiatry, 12,* 54-64.

Canadian Society for Exercise Physiology (CSEP), (2004). The Canadian physical activity, fitness and lifestyle approach (CPAFLA): CSEP health and fitness program's health-related appraisal and counseling strategy (3rd ed.). Ottawa: Author.

Carroll, D., Gleeson, C., Ribsby, B., and Dugdale, A.E. (1986). Body build and the desire for slenderness in young people. *Australian Paediatric Journal, 22,* 121-125.

Carter, J. E. L. (2002). The 2-D somatochart and X,Y coordinates. In *The Heath-Carter Anthropometric Somatotype Instruction Manual* [Web]. San Diego: Retrieved March 11, 2007, from http://www.somatotype.org/Heath-CarterManual.pdf

DiGioacchino, R. F., Sargent, R. G., and Topping, M. (2001). Body dissatisfaction among White and African American male and female college students. *Eating Behaviours, 2,* Retrieved June 30, 2006, from http://www.elsevier.com.

Dwyer, J.T., Feldman, J.J., Seltser, C.C., and Meyer, J. (1969). Adolescent attitudes toward weight and appearance. *Journal of Nutrition Education, Fall,* 14-19.

Holder, M. and Keates, J. (2006). Size of drawings influences body size estimates by women with and without eating concerns. *Body Image, 3,* Retrieved June 30, 2006 from http://www.elesvier.com.

The International Society for the Advancement in Kinanthropometry (ISAK). *International Standards for Anthropometric Assessment.* Underdale, SA, Australia: ISAK, 2001, 1-133.

Leonhard, M.L. and Barry, N.J. (1998). Body image and obesity: effects of gender and weight on perceptual measure of body image. *Addictive Behaviors, 23,* 31-34.

Malina, R.M., Bouchard, C., and Bar-Or, O. (2004). *Growth, maturation, and physical activity* (2nd ed.). Champaign, Il: Human Kinetics.

Manley, R. S., Tonkin, R., and Hammond, C. (1988). A method for the assessment of body image disturbance in patients with eating disorders. *Journal of Adolescent Health Care, 9,* 384-388.

Merriam-Webster (2002). *Merriam-Webster's Medical Dictionary.* Retrieved October 3, 2006, from Dictionary.com website: http://dictionary.reference.com/browse/body image.

Mueller, W. H., Joos, S. K., and Schull, W. J. (1985). Alternative measurements of obesity: accuracy of body silhouette and reported weights and heights in a Mexican American sample. *International Journal of Obesity, 9,* 193-200.

Rozin, P., Trachtenberg, S., and Cohen, A. B. (2001). Stability of body image and body image dissatisfaction in American college students over about the last 15 years. *Appetite, 37,* Retrieved September 27, 2006, from http://www.idealibrary.com.

Sheldon, W.H., Dupertuis, C.W., and McDermott, E. (1955). *Atlas of men: a guide for somatotyping the adult male at all ages.* New York: Harper and Brothers.

Sheldon, W.H., Stevens, S.S., and Tucker, W.B. (1940). *The varieties of human physique.* New York: Harper and Brothers.

Shih, M. and Kubo, C. (2005). Body shape preference and body satisfaction of Taiwanese and Japanese female college students. *Psychiatry Research, 133,* Retrieved September 27, 2006 from http://www.elsevier.com.

Sobral, F. and Vasconcelos, O. (1996). Perceived somatotype as indicator of accuracy of body image, a method using somatotype attitudinal distance. *Perceptual and Motor Skills, 82,* 1107-1110.

Stuhldreher, W. and Ryan, W. (1999). Factors associated with distortion in body image perception in college women. *American Journal of Health Studies, 15,* 8-12.

Stunkard, A. J., Sorenson, T., and Schulsinger, F. (1983). Use of the Danish adoption register for the study of obesity and thinness. In S. Kety (ed.), *The Genetics of Neurological and Psychiatric Disorders,* 115-120. New York: Raven Press.

Tanner, J. M. and Whitehouse, R. H. (1982). *Atlas of children's growth: normal variation and growth disorders.* London: Academic Press.

Tehard, B., Van Liere, M. J., Com Nougué, C., and Clavel-Chapelon, F. (2002). Anthropometric measurements and body silhouette of women: validity and perception. *Journal of the American Dietetic Association, 102,* 1779-1784.

Thompson, A.M. and Chad, K.E. (2000). The relationship of pubertal status to body image, social physique anxiety, preoccupation with weight and nutritional status in young females. *Canadian Journal of Public Health, 91*(3), 207-211.

Thompson, A.M. and Chad, K.E. (2005). Selected antecedent that place young females at risk for developing an eating disorder. In P.I. Swain (ed) *Adolescent Eating Disorders*, New York, Nova Science, 97-114.

Thompson, M.A. and Gray, J.J. (1995). Development and validation of a new body-image assessment scale. *Journal of Personality Assessment, 64,* 258-269.

Turner, S. L., Hamilton, H., Jacobs, M., Angood, L. M., and Dwyer, D. H. (1997). The influence of fashion magazines on the body image satisfaction of college women: an exploratory analysis. *Adolescence, 32,* 603-613.

In: Exercise and Women's Health
Editor: Laura A. Charlington, pp. 127-141
ISBN: 978-1-60456-013-8

Chapter 6

CHANGES IN PSYCHOLOGICAL WELL-BEING IN DEPRESSED WOMEN FOLLOWING A MULTI-DISCIPLINARY THERAPY PROGRAM, INCLUDING PSYCHOMOTOR THERAPY

J. Knapen*, D. Vancampfort, G. Pieters, P. Sienaert and J. Peuskens
University Psychiatric Centre K.U.Leuven, Campus Kortenberg, Leuvensesteenweg 517, 3070 Kortenberg, Belgium
Department of Rehabilitation Sciences, Faculty of Kinesiology and Rehabilitation Sciences, Katholieke Universiteit Leuven, Belgium
Departement of Neuro Sciences, Faculty of Medicine, Katholieke Universiteit Leuven, Belgium

ABSTRACT

The objective of this exploratory one-group pre-post test study was to evaluate the nature of psychological change in inward depressed psychiatric patients attending a multi-disciplinary treatment, including psychomotor therapy. Female depressed psychiatric patients ($n = 51$) were examined before and after this program over a period of 3 months. The following psychological parameters were assessed by means of self-reporting questionnaires: depression, anxiety, global self-esteem, and physical self-worth. Patients demonstrated statistically significant improvements in depression, anxiety, global self-esteem and physical self-worth ($t(50)$ ranging from -3.76 to 4.65, all $p < 0.007$; ES ranging from 0.53 to -0.65). Changes in depression and anxiety displayed a strong negative correlation with changes in global self-esteem and physical self-worth (r varying from -0.39 to -0.67). Patients with greater improvement in physical self-worth reported greater improvement in anxiety and global self-esteem then patients who did not improve physical self-worth. Consequently, within the limitations of the research design it can be concluded that the program appeared successful in improving psychological

* Corresponding author: Jan Knapen, University Psychiatric Centre K.U.Leuven, Campus Kortenberg, Leuvensesteenweg 517, 3070 Kortenberg, Belgium; e-mail: jan.knapen@faber.kuleuven.be

well-being in female depressed patients. Results also provide preliminary insight into the potential role of physical self-worth in the recovery process of depressed patients.

INTRODUCTION

Depression is acknowledged to be one of the most common mental diseases. The World Health Organization [1] estimated that 5-10% of the world population is suffering from identifiable depression and needs psychiatric treatment or psychosocial intervention. The life-time risk of developing depression is 10-20% in females and slightly less in males. Today, depression is already the second cause of the disability-adjusted life year in the age category 15-44 years for both sexes combined. By the year 2020, depression is projected to reach second place in the ranking of the disability-adjusted life year calculated for all ages, including both sexes.

According to the current diagnostic criteria for depression following the American Psychiatric Association [2] (see box I), therapeutic intervention, therefore, can no longer solely aim to relieve severity through psycho-pharmacotherapy and/or psychotherapy. This implies that patients suffering from severe depression should be treated within a multidimensional therapeutic model, focusing on the complexity of the bio-psychosocial causes and symptoms of depression.

Box I. The American Psychiatric Association criteria for diagnosis of major depressive disorder

Five (or more) of the following symptoms have been present during the same 2-week period and represent a change from previous functioning; at least one of the symptoms is either (1) depressed mood or (2) loss of interest or pleasure.

Depressed mood, nearly every day during most of the day
Marked diminished interest or pleasure in almost all activities
Significant weight loss (when not dieting), weight gain, or a change in appetite
Insomnia or hypersomnia (excess sleep)
Psychomotor agitation or psychomotor retardation
Fatigue or loss of energy
Feelings of worthlessness or inappropriate guilt
Impaired ability to concentrate or indecisiveness
Recurrent thoughts of death, recurrent suicidal ideation

Depressive disorders are associated with a high incidence of co-morbid somatic illness. Patients suffering from major depression run a higher relative risk of cardiovascular disease, diabetes and osteoporosis than the general population [3-6]. Depression is an independent risk factor for cardiovascular disease [6]. In general, depressed patients exhibit a less active life-style and have a reduced cardio-respiratory fitness in comparison with the general population [7-9]. Several symptoms of the depressive syndrome such as loss of energy, interest and motivation, and general fatigue are directly related to a more sedentary life-style, a decreased cardio-respiratory capacity and poor physical health. In these patients a vicious cycle between avoidance of exercise, deterioration of cardio-respiratory capacity and a loss of control over functioning of the body may develop [10].

In the recent decade, there has been growing attention in the research literature on physical exercise as a potential adjunctive therapy to the traditional treatments for depression. Two meta-analyses were conducted in the area of exercise and depression. The meta-analysis of Craft and Landers [11] reported that regular exercise is as beneficial as individual or group psychotherapy and other behavioural interventions for mild to moderate depressed individuals. The meta-analysis of Lawlor and Hopker [12] encompassed 14 trials using outpatients. Compared with no treatment, exercise significantly reduced symptoms of depression (Beck Depression Inventory: weighted mean difference -7.3) [13]. The effect of exercise was similar to that of cognitive therapy. In one randomized controlled trial comparing aerobic exercise, sertraline and both in combination for the treatment of depressed outpatients ($n = 156$), the three groups showed comparable remission rates at the end of 16 weeks [14]. However, the exercise group had a significantly lower relapse rate than the sertraline and the combination groups 6 months after completion of treatment [15]. Exercising on the patient's own initiative during the 6-month follow-up period was associated with a reduced probability of major depression diagnosis at the end of that period (OR 0.49; $P = 0.0009$). The latter naturally does not exclude the possibility that the least depressive patients had the greatest interest and motivation to exercise. Another randomized controlled trial was designed to test (1) whether exercise is an efficacious treatment for outpatients suffering from mild to moderate major depressive disorder, and (2) the dose-response relation of exercise and reduction in depressive symptoms [16]. Participants were randomized to one of four aerobic exercise treatment groups that varied total energy expenditure (7.0 kcal/kg/week or 17.5 kcal/kg/week) and frequency (3 days/week or 5 days/week) or to exercise placebo control (3 days/week flexibility exercise). The 17.5 kcal/kg/week dose was consistent with public health recommendations for physical activity. The study demonstrated that aerobic exercise at public health dose is an effective treatment for major depressive disorder of mild to moderate severity (mean reduction in Hamilton Rating Scale for Depression: 47%) [17]. The effect of the lower dose was only comparable to the placebo effect (mean reduction: 30% and 29%, respectively). The exercise frequency (3 days/week versus 5 days/week) did not influence the effect on depression reduction.

There are different hypothesized mechanisms by which exercise is thought to influence depression [18]. Several physiological mechanisms such as the monoamine hypothesis, the endorphin hypothesis and the thermo-genesis hypothesis as well as psychological mechanisms such as the distraction hypothesis and the mastery and self-esteem hypothesis have been suggested. To date, research supporting physiological explanations has been weak, with many studies being poorly designed. While psychologically based explanations, specifically the mastery and self-esteem models have had consistent empirical support. One such model is the Exercise and Self-Esteem Model of Sonstroem and Morgan [19], which is based on the self-efficacy theory of Bandura [20]. This model assumes that involvement in physical activity increases physical ability, which positively influences one's self-estimation and consequently leads to higher physical self-worth.

The Exercise and Self-Esteem Model

Low self-esteem is closely related to mental illness such as clinical depression, anxiety disorders and personality disorders [2,21,22]. Most recently, Beck et al. [22], and Van de Vliet et al. [23] have indicated an inverse relationship between level of self-esteem and severity of depression and anxiety in sample groups of psychiatric outpatients and inpatients, respectively. The latter also detected that Flemish depressed psychiatric inpatients had significantly lower self-esteem and physical self-concept when compared with non-patients. A prospective study suggested that low self-esteem may play a causal role in major depressive disorders [24]. Improvement of self-esteem has therefore regularly been described as one of the main treatment aims for depressed psychiatric patients. Fox [21] considers self-esteem to be the affective component of the self director, defining it as 'A self-rating of how well the self is doing'. Campbell [25] defines self-esteem as 'An awareness of good possessed by self'. Self-concept is considered to be the cognitive component of the self director [21]. It is a multidimensional self-description, which contains more specific perceptions in different constructs. These constructs are therefore regarded as components or domains of the global self-concept. Roles in several life domains may contribute to the global self-concept and include perceptions of the self at work or in school (academic self-concept), in social relationships (social self-concept), in emotional relationships (emotional self-concept), and also perceptions about the body and physical abilities (physical self-concept). Physical self-concept is dictated by qualities related to physical acceptance and physical competence [21]. During the last twenty years, much value has been attached to body attractiveness, health-related physical fitness, motor skills and sporting performances as these features of the physical domain are consistently tied to the global self-concept. As a result, the physical self-concept may be important for the development and the enhancement of global self-concept especially for individuals with low self-concept such as psychiatric patients. Leith [26] indicated that clinical populations in particular (e.g. depressed adults, persons with mental retardation, rehabilitation patients) have problems with self-concept. He also reported that exercise programs lead to a significant improvement in self-concept in 77% of the conducted investigations with these groups. He also reported that exercise programs lead to a significant improvement in self-concept in ten out of thirteen conducted investigations with these groups. The 'Exercise and Self-Esteem Model', developed by Sonstroem and Morgan [19] and further by Fox [27] represents the theoretical framework of the hierarchical model of self-concept. This model proposes that physical self-perceptions can be improved through physical activity participation. Improvements in specific physical self-perceptions (e.g. stamina, muscular strength, attractiveness of body) may generalize to physical self-worth in general. In turn, physical self-worth is related to global self-esteem. Finally, increased global self-esteem can lead to a reduction of depression and anxiety.

In depressed patients, a low physical self-concept and poor physical health and fitness, in interaction with other barriers to participation in exercise, such as psychosomatic complaints and hypochondria, lack of energy, and general fatigue may lead to a vicious cycle of loss of self-confidence, an increased avoidance of physical activity and decreased levels of physical health and fitness [10]. For that reason, the incorporation of exercise therapy into the comprehensive treatment programs for depressed patients is highly recommended. During the last three decades research findings in the area of physical activity and mental and physical health has led to an 'evidence-based' implementation of physical exercise as psychomotor therapy in many psychiatric hospitals [28].

Study Objectives

The present study is a pre-experimental investigation that aims at the description of the nature of changes in depression, anxiety, global self-esteem and physical self-worth in female depressed patients attending a multi-disciplinary program, including psychomotor therapy, over a period of 3 months. It was hypothesized that depression and anxiety symptoms are reduced and global self-esteem and physical self-worth improved through the multi-modal therapeutic program.

The second aim of the present study addresses the relationship between physical self-worth, global self-esteem, depression and anxiety. We assumed that participation in psychomotor therapy involving three exercise sessions per week successfully improves patient's physical self-worth. As physical self-worth is a key component of the global self-esteem [21] it was hypothesized therefore that improvements in physical self-worth are related to improvements in global self-esteem, depression and anxiety.

METHOD

Participants

Participants were consecutive female patients with a major depressive disorder [2] and an elevated depression score (Beck Depression Inventory > 15) [13], recruited from the cognitive-behavioural wards of a university psychiatric hospital in Belgium. In the first week of admission, patients were asked to take part in the study. Evaluations were performed the first week of admission and after three months treatment. Patients were excluded from the investigation in cases of: (1) bipolar disorders, (2) psychotic episodes, (3) somatic contra-indications for physical exercise (e.g. severe cardiovascular, neuromuscular and/or orthopaedic diseases). In many cases trained psychiatrists reported an underlying diagnosis of personality disorders (e.g. borderline, histrionic, avoidant or dependent personality disorders) [2]. Most patients were on a stable antidepressant regimen at an adequate dosage for at least 6-8 weeks prior to inclusion and they continued pharmacological treatment without changes throughout the trial. The final sample was 51 female patients (mean age: 33.42 ± 10.58 years). The study was approved by the Ethical Committee of the Faculty of Medicine of the Katholieke Universiteit Leuven. Written informed consent was obtained from all patients before entering the study.

Treatment Program

Patients followed a multi-disciplinary cognitive-behavioural therapy program. It included: psycho-pharmacotherapy, psychiatric consultation, individual cognitive-behavioural therapy, different forms of group psychotherapy and social skill training, partner or family therapy, occupational therapy, leisure time supervision and fitness training as psychomotor therapy. Details of the comprehensive treatment program are described in Knapen et al. [29].

Psychomotor Therapy

The physical fitness program was a combination of aerobic and muscular fitness training three times a week. Each session lasted 45 minutes and consisted of a warming-up with stretching exercises, an exercise phase and a cooling-down phase including repeated stretching. The exercise units were the treadmill, the multi-station resistance machine, the rowing machine, the bicycle ergo-meter, the cross-trainer and the step machine. Depending on the outcome of the initial fitness assessments, the participant's own expectations and goals, and earlier experiences with physical training, the psychomotor therapists developed a gradual exercise program by applying the general recommendations of the American College of Sports Medicine [30]. The work load of aerobic training was moderate, since more intensive effort is associated with greater cardio-vascular risk, orthopedic injury and lower adherence to training on account of higher perceived exertion and discomfort. The relative intensity, measured by heart rate monitors, ranged from 40% to 60% of the estimated maximal heart rate reserve following Karvonen [31]. Perceived exertion, rated by the Borg Category Ratio 10 Scale, was used as an adjunct for the intensity prescription at each exercise apparatus [32]. The rate of perceived exertion, especially in clinical populations, is a valuable aid in teaching participants to monitor exercise tolerance taking account of their own level of fatigue, rate of breathing and muscular sensations. For most patients, the intensity of effort corresponded to a value of 3-4 (moderate to somewhat strong) on the Borg Category Ratio 10 Scale. The duration of the exercise bouts, 5-10 minutes at the beginning of the program, was prolonged to approximately 20 minutes before the work load was increased. The dynamic resistance training constituted a well-rounded program exercising all major muscle groups. Muscular strength and endurance were developed by the progressive overload principle according to which repetitions and weight load are gradually increased. Generally, the number of repetitions in each exercise set was 10-15, since a lower frequency at a higher intensity increases blood pressure and the risk of orthopedic injury in subjects with a low initial muscular fitness. The number of exercise sets (one to three) depended on the level of the participant's muscular fitness, the goals she wished to achieve, and on the time available for each workout. The program was monitored using exercise cards and the patients were informed regularly about their progress by the psychomotor therapists. The therapists avoided between-patient comparisons. Participants and therapist discussed their experiences with the exercises during the last five minutes of each session. Discussions were focused on personal experiences with the exercises (e.g. sense of mastery, stress reduction, enjoyment and satisfaction) and on body awareness (e.g. breathing, muscle tone and relaxation, degree of effort, body-acceptance). The program was based on mastery experiences, personal responsibility, social reinforcement, self-evaluation, constructive feedback by therapist, hedonic properties of exercise and process internalization [33].

Measures

Questionnaires were administered to assess depression, anxiety, global self-esteem and physical self-worth. All questionnaires were already available and tested on psychometric properties in the Dutch language at the time of administration.

The Beck Depression Inventory

The Beck Depression Inventory (BDI) [34] is a 21-item self-reporting questionnaire consisting of symptoms and attitudes relating to depression. The range of possible total scores is 0-63 with higher scores indicate greater depression. The Dutch version of the BDI has been shown to be a valid and reliable measure of depression severity [34]. Internal consistency measure in the present study was 0.77.

Trait Anxiety Inventory

The Trait Anxiety Inventory (TAI) subscale of the State-Trait Anxiety Inventories (STAI) [35] was used to assess trait anxiety. This self-rating scale that consists of 20 items, with response scores on a scale from 1 to 4. The range of possible total scores is 20-80; higher score indicate higher levels of anxiety. The TAI represents one of the most reliable and valid instruments for assessing trait anxiety in psychiatric settings, and has been validated for use in Dutch by Hermans [35]. Internal consistency measure of the TAI-subscale in the present study was 0.89.

The Rosenberg Self-Esteem Scale (RSES)

The RSES [36] was used to evaluate global self-esteem and self-acceptance. This self-rating scale is composed of 10 items. Higher total scores indicate higher self-esteem (range: 10-40). The Dutch version of the RSES is regarded as one of the better measures of global self-esteem [36]. The internal consistency measure in the present study was 0.86.

The Physical Self-Perception Profile

Physical self-concept was assessed using the domain scale of Physical Self-Worth (PSW) in the Dutch version of the Physical Self-Perception Profile (PSPP) [23]. This version of the PSPP consists of the domain scale of PSW (6 items: general feelings of happiness, satisfaction, pride, respect and confidence in the physical self) and three specific sub-domain scales, namely perception of sports competence and physical condition, perceived attractive body and perceived physical strength. Each item is scored on a scale from 1 to 4, with higher scores indicating more positive self-perceptions. The range of possible total scores for the PSW scale is 0-24. Van de Vliet et al [23] demonstrated an adequate reliability and validity of The Dutch version of the PSPP in a sample group of Flemish psychiatric inpatients. Internal consistency measure of the physical self-worth scale in the present study was 0.93.

Statistical Analysis

Data analysis included calculating paired t-tests for examining differences between before and after treatment measures for all variables, including Bonferroni correction for multiple testing problems. Effect sizes were calculated as the mean score before treatment was subtracted from the mean score after treatment, and divided with the standard deviation of the difference score [ES = (M_{after} M_{before})/$SD_{difference}$) [37]. As a general guideline, an ES of 0.20 to 0.50 is considered a small effect, 0.50 to 0.80 medium and greater than 0.80 large.

Relationships between changes in outcome variables were examined with Pearson product-moment correlation coefficients.

Based on the relative changes in physical self-worth between pre- and post measure, the group of subjects was therefore split into four groups using the quartile method. Each subject was classified as either having experienced a large improvement (n = 13), a moderate improvement (n=14), no improvement or a moderate decline (n = 14), or a large decline (n = 14). With respect to comparison between groups with different initial depression profiles, a categorization was made into subgroups with mild to moderate depression (16-19), moderate to severe depression (20-29), and severe depression (BDI > 29), following the criteria set by Beck et al. [13]. Analysis of variance and Tukey post hoc tests were used to compare the different groups. The statistical significance level was set at 0.05 (two-tailed). All analyses were performed using Statistica 5.5 [38].

RESULTS

As expected, initial mean depression score indicated the presence of moderate to severe depression level. Trait anxiety level was also elevated, indicating widespread presence of trait anxiety symptoms. Measures of global self-esteem and physical self-worth were significantly lower than scores of non-depressed women (table 1, columns 7-8, t-values -12.00 and -10.8, both $p < 0.01$; measures taken from Van de Vliet et al. [23]).

Changes in Depression, Anxiety, Global Self-Esteem and Physical Self-Worth after 3 Months of Therapeutic Intervention

Table 1 shows the descriptive statistics for all variables before and after the three-month therapeutic intervention period, as well as the difference scores (M_{after} M_{before}).

Depressed women reported lower depression and anxiety levels ($t(50) = 4.65$, $p < 0.007$, ES = -0.65 for depression and $t(50) = 3.95$, $p < 0.007$, ES = -0.55 for trait anxiety); and significant improvements in global self-esteem and physical self-worth ($t(50) = -3.76$, $p < 0.007$, ES = 0.53 for global self-esteem and $t(50)$ -3.95, $p < 0.007$, ES = 0.55 for physical self-worth) were found after 3 months of treatment. These results represented moderate effect sizes.

With respect to the categories of depression, provided by Beck et al. [13], twenty-eight patients (55%) decreased their depression level by the end of the program. Eighteen patients (35%) did not change category. Only five patients (10%) increased their depression level.

Changes in physical self-worth were related significantly to changes in global self-esteem, depression and anxiety in the expected direction (r ranging from -0.39 to -0.50, all $p < 0.01$).

Table 1. Descriptive statistics and differences (mean ± standard deviation) before and after treatment for depression, anxiety, global self-esteem and physical self-worth in female depressed psychiatric patients (n = 51) (t-test, ES); comparison with healthy women (data derived from Van de Vliet et al., 2002)

Variable	Before treatment	After treatment	Difference score (Mafter – Mbefore)	t-test (df)	ES	Van de Vliet et al.	t-test (df)
Depression	28.71 ± 8.77	21.55 ±14.02	-7.16 ± 10.99	4.65 (50)*	-0.65		
Anxiety	62. 63 ± 7.19	55.51 ± 13.63	-7.12 ± 12.87	3.95 (50)*	-0.55		
Global self-esteem	21.06 ± 5.55	24.25 ± 6.79	3.20 ± 6.06	-3.76 (50)*	0.53	31.25 ± 4.40 (n=124)	-12.00 (173)**
Physical self-worth	9.67 ± 2.73	12.08 ± 4.03	2.41 ± 4.36	-3.95 (50)*	0.55	14.30 ± 3.16 (n=154)	-10.08 (203)**

*p < 0.007 (Bonferroni correction)
**p < 0.01 (Bonferroni correction).

Table 2. Changes in depression, anxiety and global self-esteem depending of the changes in physical self-worth (incl. post hoc comparison)

VARIABLE	1. Large improvement (n=13)	2. Moderate improvement (n=14)	3. No improvement/ moderate worsening (n=14)	4. Worsening (n=10)	ANOVA *F*(3.47)
Δ BDI	-12.62 ± 7.50	-9.07 ± 15.03	-3.00 ± 8.03	-3.20 ± 9.16	2.52
Δ TAI	-16.08 ± 14.22	-8.21 ± 10.39	-0.07 ± 11.38	-3.80 ± 10.04	4.55* (1 vs. 3)
Δ RSE	7.54 ± 7.01	4.43 ± 4.77	0.93 ± 4.71	-1.00 ± 4.08	6.09* (1 vs. 3,4)

*p<0.017 (Bonferroni correction)
(Δ BDI: change in depression; Δ TAI: change in trait anxiety; Δ RSE: change in global self-esteem).

The data in table 2, finally, compare the reduction of depressive and anxiety symptoms and the improvement in global self-esteem in the four groups with different profile of change in physical self-worth. The group with a large improvement in physical self-worth reported significantly greater improvement in trait anxiety and global self-esteem than those patients who do not improve or decline in physical self-worth (post hoc $p < 0.015$).

CONCLUSION

Limitations of the Study

Before discussing the results, the limitations of the present study need to be addressed. At first, the present investigation was a pre-experimental investigation. According to Thomas and Nelson [39] this is a weak research design. Accordingly, the interpretation of the data from the present study is limited. It was however the aim of the authors to explore changes in psychological well-being in a natural (therapeutic) setting without interruption of the therapeutic process. The present findings do not allow the full determination of the effectiveness of the therapy. It is not possible to compare the present data to the effects of spontaneous recovery from depression in severely depressed women in absence of a no-treatment control group. Furthermore, figures on the course of recovery during follow-up are not available.

Main Findings

Despite the absence of a non-treatment control group, the results suggest that more than two-thirds of the patients were successful in decreasing their depressive symptoms over a relatively short period of time. However, it should be stressed that patients were treated in tertiary care. They have failed to recovery after help in the primary and secondly care system, so expectations should be realistic. Evaluation of the intake profiles of the participants of the present study indicate that the diagnosis of major depressive disorder often goes along with an underlying personality disorder and a complexity of psychological, social and somatic maladjustment or problems. Besides that, a number of patients will cognitively minimize their condition (leading to under-scoring or over-scoring on the self-reporting questionnaires at onset), while during therapy they arrive at admitting the seriousness of their problems. This phenomenon of negation and overestimation is well-described in the cognitive-behavioural treatment of depressed patients [40]. The outcome, however, is expressed by a `worsening' of their scores.

Participants Were Not Volunteers for Exercise

In contrast with many other investigations in the field of exercise and psychological well-being using non-clinical volunteers [12], patients were not 'selected' and all of them were sequentially referred to the study. Patients were not volunteers for exercise, considering that they initially sought treatment to discuss psychological ailments and to ask for assistance with their social problems, usually expecting a psychopharmacological and psychotherapeutic treatment. At onset of treatment, most depressed patients tended to be passive receivers. Psychomotor therapy, which appeals to the patient's own active participation and responsibility, does initially not meet their immediate needs. It is therefore reasonable to assume that the compliance and effectiveness with exercise in depressed patients would be worse than in the general population. Many depressed patients demonstrate multiple risk factors for non-compliance in exercise programs, such as learned helplessness, hypochondria, a loss of energy and interest, smoking, general fatigue, a negative physical self-concept, a low intrinsic motivation and poor physical health and fitness [7,12,41,42]. Despite these psychological and physical barriers to participate in exercise, there was a good adherence to the intervention. This may be attributable to the motivational strategies and the supportive and task-oriented climate put into place by the psychomotor therapists [43]. It is plausible that in psychomotor therapy for depressed patients, certain elements are critical to ensuring optimal exercise adherence, allowing physical self-concept enhancement to take place. These elements are (1) an enhanced body acceptance and perceived physical competence (2) goal achievement (3) self-evaluation, social reinforcement and constructive feedback by therapist (4) an enhanced sense of personal control over the body and its functioning (5) an improved sense of belonging and social significance through relationships with peers (6) self-determination (7) focus on personal responsibility and hedonic properties of exercise [21,33]. Every effort was made to implement all these mechanisms in the program.

The mean score of the physical self-worth has been increased after 3 months intervention however it is acceptable that not all patients experienced positive effects on physical self-concept. One possible explanation for this is that a large number of patients suffered from recurrent depressive disorders, often associated with an underlying complex personality disorder. In most cases, these patients had failed to recover in treatment in primary and/or secondary care. They were characterized by persistent feelings of incompetence and failure, and overestimation, overgeneralization and internal attributions with regard to negative events. Many of them exhibited low self-acceptance or high self-criticism and were therefore unable to reach their (unrealistic) expectations. A second explanation for not experiencing progress in physical self-concept is related to the barriers to exercise participation that depressed patients experience [7,41,42].

Relationship between Changes in Outcome Variables

The second aim of the present study was to identify the relationship between physical self-worth, global self-esteem, depression and anxiety. Improvements in physical self-worth went along with an increase in global self-esteem and a decline in depression and anxiety levels. This finding corroborates the Exercise and Self-Esteem Model [19,27], which is based on the self-efficacy theory of Bandura [20]. This hierarchical model proposes that improvements in physical self-concept lead to enhancements in global self-esteem. In turn, increased global self-esteem can lead to a reduction of depression and anxiety. The founded relationships provide some interesting information regarding the potential role of the physical self in the recovery process of depressed women. However, it also remains possible that changes in depression, anxiety and/or global self-esteem improve a subject's physical self-worth.

Benefits of Physical Fitness

The fact that exercise is associated with physical health benefits and fitness gains (depressed patients have poor physical health and low physical fitness), as well as with psychological benefits is an important argument for the incorporation of psychomotor therapy into treatment programs for depressed patients [3-9]. In our sample group, participation in psychomotor therapy resulted in an improvement of cardio-respiratory fitness (13.59% increase in physical work capacity) as well as in muscular strength [10].

Exercise as Health Promotion in the General Population

According to a report of the World Health Organization [44], at least 60% of the global population fails to achieve the minimum recommendation for health-related physical fitness (i.e., 30 minutes moderate intensity physical activity daily). Regular physical exercise is significantly less common in women than in men and significantly less among those older than 44. The relationship between lack of regular physical activity and depression in both middle-aged and older women has been the subject of two prospective cohort studies. The study of Brown [45] examined the dose-response relationship between self-reported physical activity and depressive symptoms in a cohort of 9.207 middle-aged women, corrected for pre-existing psychological and physical health problems. The data suggested that there is a clear dose-response relationship between increasing physical activity and decreasing depressive symptoms, independent of pre-existing physical and psychological health. Lee and Russell [46] reported on the longitudinal effects of physical activity and psychological well-being among older Australian women. Overall, women who had become physically active over a 3 year interval had positive changes in psychological well-being, while the opposite was true in those who had become less active. Due to the relationships between physical activity, physical fitness, and treatment and prevention of depression and co-morbid diseases (i.e. cardiovascular disease, diabetes and osteoporosis) the promotion of physical activity may be a feasible physical and mental health promotion strategy. A variety of community interventions exist that are able to increase physical activity in the general population. The effectiveness of such interventions also needs to be evaluated in terms of preventing depression.

References

[1] World Health Organization: *Prevention of Mental Disorders: Effective Interventions and Policy Option: Summary Report.* Geneva, World Health Organization, 2004.

[2] American Psychiatric Association: *Diagnostic and Statistical Manual of Mental Disorders,* ed 4. Washington, American Psychiatric Association, 1994.

[3] Fenton W, Stover E: Mood disorders. Cardiovascular and diabetes comorbidity. *Curr Opin Psychiatry* 2006;19:421-7.

[4] Kahl K, Greggersen W, Rudolf S, Stoeckelhuber B, Bergmann-Koester C, Dibbelt L, Schweiger U: Bone mineral density, bone turnover, and osteoprotegerin in depressed women with and without borderline personality disorder. *Psychosom. Med.* 2006;68:669-74.

[5] Whooley M: Depression and cardiovascular disease. Healing the broken-hearted. *JAMA*. 2006;295:2874-81.

[6] Lett H, Blumenthal J, Babyak M, Sherwood A, Strauman T, Robins C, Newman M: Depression as a risk factor for coronary artery disease: Evidence, mechanisms, and treatment. *Psychosom. Med.* 2004;66:305-15.

[7] Meyer T, Broocks A: Therapeutic impact of exercise on psychiatric diseases: Guidelines for exercise testing and prescription. *Sports. Med.* 2000;30:269-79.

[8] Knapen J, Van de Vliet P, Van Coppenolle H, Peuskens J, Pieters G: Evaluation of cardio-respiratory fitness and perceived exertion for patients with depressive and anxiety disorders: A study on reliability. *Disabil. Rehabil.* 2003;25:1312-5.

[9] Hollenberg M, Haight T, Tager I: Depression decreases cardiorespiratory fitness in older women. *J. Clin. Epidemiol.* 2003;56:1111-7.

[10] Knapen J, Van de Vliet P, Van Coppenolle H, David A, Peuskens J, Knapen K, Pieters G: Improvements in physical fitness of non-psychotic psychiatric patients following psychomotor therapy programs. *J. Sports Med. Phys. Fitness.* 2003;43:513-22.

[11] Craft L, Landers D: The effect of exercise on clinical depression and depression resulting from mental illness: A meta-analysis. *J. Sport Exerc. Psychol.* 1998;20:339-57.

[12] Lawlor D, Hopker, S: The effectiveness of exercise as an intervention in the management of depression: Systematic review and meta-regression analysis of randomised controlled trials. *BMJ.* 2001;322:763-7.

[13] Beck A, Steer R, Garbin M: Psychometric properties of the Beck Depression Inventory: Twenty-five years of evaluation. *Clin. Psychol. Rev.* 1988;8:77-100.

[14] Blumenthal J, Babyak M, Moore K, Craighead W, Herman S, Khatri P, Waugh R, Napolitano M, Forman L, Appelbaum M, Doraiswamy M, Krishnan K: Effects of exercise training on older patients with major depression. *Arch. Intern. Med.* 1999;159:2349-56.

[15] Babyak M, Blumenthal J, Herman S, Khatri P, Doraiswamy M, Moore K, Craighead W, Baldewicz T, Krishnan K: Exercise treatment for major depression: maintenance of therapeutic benefit at 10 months. *Psychosom. Med.* 2000;62:633-8.

[16] Dunn A, Trivedi M, Kampert J, Clark C, Chambliss H: Exercise treatment for depression: Efficacy and dose response. *Am. J. Prev. Med.* 2005;28:1-8.

[17] Hamilton M: A rating scale for depression. *J. Neurol. Neurosurg. Psychiatry.* 1960;23:56-62.

[18] Daley A: Exercise therapy and mental health in clinical populations: is exercise therapy a worthwhile intervention? *Advances in Psychiatric Treatment.* 2002;8:262-70.

[19] Sonstroem R, Morgan W: Exercise and self-esteem: Rationale and model. *Med. Sci. Sports Exerc.* 1989;21:329-37.

[20] Bandura A: Self-efficacy: Towards a unifying theory of behavior change. *Psychol. Rev.* 1977;84:191-215.

[21] Fox K: Self-esteem, self-perceptions and exercise. *Int. J. Sport Psychol.* 2000;31:228-40.

[22] Beck A, Brown G, Steer R, Kuyken W, Grisham J: Psychometric properties of the Beck Self-Esteem Scales. *Behav. Res. Ther.* 2001;39:115-24.

[23] Van de Vliet P, Knapen J, Onghena P, Fox K, Van Coppenolle H, David A, Pieters G, Peuskens J: Assessment of physical self-perceptions in normal Flemish adults versus depressed psychiatric patients. *Pers. Individ. Dif.* 2002;32:855-63.

[24] Maciejewski P: Self-efficacy as a mediator between stressful life events and depressive symptoms: differences based on history of prior depression. *Br. J. Psychiatry.* 2000;176:373-8.

[25] Campbell R: *The New Science: Self-Esteem Psychology.* Lanham, University Press of America, 1984.

[26] Leith L: *Foundations of Exercise and Mental Health.* Morgantown, Fitness Information Technology, 1994.

[27] Fox K: The physical self and processes in self-esteem development; in Fox K (ed): *The Physical Self: From Motivation to Well-Being.* Champaign, Human Kinetics, 1997, pp 111-140.

[28] Knapen J, Van de Vliet P, Van Coppenolle H, David A, Peuskens J, Pieters G, Knapen K: Comparison of changes in physical self-concept, global self-esteem, depression and anxiety following two different psychomotor therapy programs in non-psychotic psychiatric inpatients. *Psychother Psychosom.* 2005;74:353-61.

[29] Knapen J, Vermeersch J, Van Coppenolle H, Cuykx V, Pieters G, Peuskens J: The physical self-concept in patients with depressive and anxiety disorders. *Int. J. Ther. Rehabil.* 2007;14:30-5.

[30] Pollock M, Gaesser G, Butcher J, Després J, Dishman R, Franklin B, Garber C: The recommended quantity and quality of exercise for developing and maintaining cardiorespiratory and muscular fitness, flexibility in healthy adults. *Med. Sci. Sports Exerc.* 1998;30:975-91.

[31] American College of Sports Medicine (US). *A.C.S.M.'s Guidelines for Exercise Testing and Prescription,* ed 6. Baltimore, Williams and Wilkins, 2000.

[32] Borg G: External, physiological and psychological factors and perceived exertion; in Borg G (ed): *Borg's Perceived Exertion and Pain Scales.* Champaign, Human Kinetics, 1998, pp 68-74.

[33] Sonstroem R: Improving compliance with exercise programs; in Torg J, Shephard R (eds): *Current Therapy in Sports Medicine.* St. Louis, Mosby, 1995, pp 608-19.

[34] Bosscher R, Koning H, van Meurs R: Reliability and validity of the Beck Depression Inventory in a Dutch college population. *Psychol. Rep.* 1986;8:696-8.

[35] Hermans D: De 'Zelf-Beoordelings-Vragenlijst' [The State-Trait Anxiety Inventory]. *Gedragstherapie.* 1994;27:145-8.

[36] Helbing J: Zelfwaardering: Meting en validiteit [Self-esteem: Measurement and validity]. *Nederlands Tijdschrift voor de Psychologie.* 1982;37:257-77.

[37] Cohen J: *Statistical Analysis for the Behavioural Sciences,* ed 2. Hillsdale, Lawrence Erlbaum,1988.

[38] Statsoft, Inc: *Statistica for Windows (computer programme).* Tulsa, Statsoft Inc, 1995.

[39] Thomas J, Nelson J: *Research Methods in Physical Activity*, ed 2. Champaign, Human Kinetics, 1996.

[40] Weismann M: Psychotherapy in the maintenance treatment of depression. *Brit. J. Psychiatry.* 1994;165:42-60.

[41] Biddle S, Mutrie N: *Psychology of Physical Activity. Determinants, Well-being and Interventions.* London, Routledge, 2001.

[42] Salmon P: Effects of physical exercise on anxiety, depression, and sensitivity to stress: A unifying theory. *Clin. Psychol. Rev.* 2001;21:33-61.

[43] Weinberg R, Gould D: *Foundations of Sport and Exercise Psychology*, ed 3. Champaign, Human Kinetics, 2003.

[44] World Health Organization: *World Health Report 2002 - Reducing Risks, Promoting Healthy Life.* Geneva, World Health Organization, 2002.

[45] Brown W, Ford J, Burton N, Marshall A, Dobson A: Prospective study of physical activity and depressive symptoms in middle-aged women. *Am. J. Prev. Med.* 2005;29:265-72.

[46] Lee C, Russell A: Prospective study of physical activity and depressive symptoms in middle-aged women. *J. Psychosom. Res.* 2003;54:155-60.

In: Exercise and Women's Health
Editor: Laura A. Charlington, pp. 143-155
ISBN: 978-1-60456-013-8

Chapter 7

PHYSICAL ACTIVITY, HEALTH AND PREVALENCE OF OVERWEIGHT AND MUSCULOSKELETAL COMPLAINTS IN YOUNG WOMEN

***Marie Alricsson*[*1] *and Debra Domalewski*[2]**
[1] Department of Health Sciences, Mid Sweden University, Östersund, Sweden;
[2] Disability and Rehabilitation Research Unit, Griffith University, Logan Campus, Brisbane, Australia.

ABSTRACT

This chapter discusses research regarding the area of physical activity, self-related health and the prevalence of overweight and body complaints in young women. The chapter integrates the results of a newly published Swedish investigation, and unpublished data from Norwegian and Australian studies regarding these topics.

It is generally accepted that physical activity provides benefits to health, functional ability and general quality of life. Physical activity also facilitates the development of motor skills and increases energy expenditure. Conversely, physical inactivity is a major public health challenge in the developed world and is recognized as a global epidemic. Furthermore, physical inactivity has emerged as an important risk factor for many chronic diseases as it has been shown to be closely related to an increased risk of cardiovascular disease, diabetes mellitus, osteoporosis and certain types of cancer. Therefore, participation in regular physical activity is important for improved bodily function and development. Unfortunately, levels of physical activity declines as young people mature, particularly among young women. European boys of all ages participate in more physical activity than European girls and the gender difference is more marked when vigorous activity is considered.

The most common argument is that young people's lack of participation in sport and physical activity is directly equated with a dramatic rise in childhood obesity. Accumulated evidence suggests that overweight youths become overweight adults, and inactive youths also become inactive adults.

---

* Correspondence concerning this chapter should be addressed to: Marie Alricsson, PhD, RPT. E-mail: marie.alricsson@miun.se

Musculoskeletal symptoms are present early in school-age and it has been suggested that these early symptoms might represent the start of a lifelong course of musculoskeletal complaints. The prevalence of the various definitions of low back pain increased greatly in the early teen years, earlier for girls than for boys. By the ages of 18 years for girls and 20 years for boys, more than 50 % had experienced at least one low back pain episode. There is a general tendency for more young women to report low back pain than young men.

Previous studies have shown that walking and cycling to school are associated with higher physical activity levels therefore correlating that active travel to school provides an opportunity for daily physical activity. Furthermore, schools should provide opportunities for young women to participate in a wider range of activities such as dancing, gymnastics, aerobics etc. to increase their physical activity and improve their health.

INTRODUCTION

In many Western countries, children and adolescents are becoming less physically active and are adopting a sedentary life-style in front of screens such as televisions, computer monitors, cinema screens or video games [1]. It is generally accepted that physical activity provides benefits to health, functional ability and general quality of life. Physical activity also facilitates the development of motor skills and increases energy expenditure. Furthermore, physical activity is additionally associated with several health outcomes in adults such as lower all-cause mortality, cardiovascular disease, some cancers, diabetes mellitus, and depressive symptoms may contribute to a lower risk of obesity and osteoporosis [2, 4-10].

Therefore, physical inactivity is a major public health challenge in the developed world and is recognized as a global epidemic [3]. Furthermore, it has been reported that physical inactivity during growth might lead to impaired health later on in life [12]. In addition to the risk posed by inactivity, some girls (the study referred to Italian girls aged 11-15 years old) are also exposed to the risks of excessive physical training from an early age, which may have an impact on growth, reproductive function and bone mineralization [11].Therefore, regular and correct participation in physical activity is important for improved bodily function and development. Unfortunately, levels of physical activity falls as young people become older, particularly among young women [12]. European boys of all ages participate in more physical activity than European girls and the gender difference is more marked when vigorous activity is considered. The physical activity levels of both genders are higher during childhood and decline as young people move through their teen years [13].

The most common argument is that young people's lack of participation in sport and physical activity is directly equated with a dramatic rise in childhood obesity. Given that physical activity is an important factor related to weight control, there is renewed interest in the relationship between physical activity and the body composition of adolescents, as well as the importance of physical activity in maintaining good health and well-being [14-15]. Sallis et al.'s research investigated the reviews of nine studies using standardized self-reports of objective measures of physical activity and identified that males are about 15 to 25 % more active than females [16]. Furthermore, during school age, a consistent decline in physical activity has been noted, with males decreasing about 2.7 % per year and females about 7.4 % per year. This data suggests that older youths and females are at increased risk of obesity due to their sedentary lifestyle [16]. Accumulated evidence also suggests that overweight youths become overweight adults, and inactive youths also become inactive adults [17-20].

However, active young women do attach significant meaning to physical activity as a space for leisure, and use it to enhance their health and well-being [21]. Weight management, social interaction, enjoyment and a slim body shape motivate participation in sport and physical activity among young women [3]. This is important in light of the fact that standardized values (e.g., metabolic rate) are often applied for estimation of energy expenditure when other, more accurate techniques (e.g., regression equations developed for the population of interest) may be more appropriate, depending on the research question).

Physical Activity

Physical activity has been defined as “any bodily movement produced by skeletal muscles that result in energy expenditure” [22]. Energy expenditure varies considerably among girls performing the same activity; an activity that may contribute significantly to daily energy expenditure in some girls will be less effective in others [23]. Expert committees have produced guidelines for health-related physical activity for youths but they are evidence-informed rather than evidence-based and were there is evidence of a relationship between physical activity during youth and health status there is little evidence showing the nature of that relationship. The number of children who experience physical activity of the duration, frequency and intensity recommended by expert committees decreases with age but accurate estimates of how many girls and boys are inactive are clouded by methodological problems such as different measurements, samples etc.

During the last decade, there has been an emphasis on what are the correct recommendations for physical activity in daily life [24]. There is a growing awareness that research is required that explores how the activity level of adolescents and their body composition are related and how that translates to the development and maintenance of a healthy body [25].

A decade ago, the International Consensus Conference in the USA on Physical Activity Guidelines for Adolescents convened to review the effects of physical activity on the health of adolescents. This meeting of delegates established age-appropriate physical activity guidelines, and considered how such guidelines could be implemented in primary health care settings. Thirty-four invited experts representing scientific, medical, and governmental organizations established two main guidelines [26]. Firstly, all adolescents should be physically active daily or nearly every day as part of their lifestyle. Secondly, adolescents should be engaged in three or more sessions per week of activities that last 20 minutes or more and that requires medium to vigorous levels of exertion [26].

In 2006 a national consensus report from Australia and New Zealand regarding monitoring and examination of physical activity in children and young people was published [27]. The project related to an identified priority in “Be active Australia: a framework for health sector activity for physical activity 2005-2010” [27]. This priority has been endorsed by the Australian Health Ministers Council [27]. Physical activity recommendations from the national consensus workshop for children and young people aged 12-18 years were to engage in vigorous activity three to four days a week for a minimum period of at least 20 minutes.

The vigorous activity recommendation is similar to the corresponding element in the adult guidelines.

The Norwegian physical activity recommendations for children and youth went a step further, stating that there should be a minimum of 60 minutes of medium intensity physical activity every day [28]. Klasson-Heggebo and Anderssen evaluated the level of physical activity in a representative cohort of urban children and youths in Norway, and identified that 86 % of 9-year-olds and 55 % of 15-year-olds met these recommendations. Furthermore, the activity level was higher among boys than girls of both age groups [28]. Supporting these findings other authors have reported that 61% to 72 % of adolescents in the same age group as above participated in physical activity [29-30]. General epidemiological findings concerning physical activity in young individuals have suggested, that boys were more active than girls, and that the amount of physical activity declined with increased age, but the rate of decline was greater in girls than boys [28, 31]. In males, a decrease was found in time spent in extremely vigorous activities, whereas in females time spent in this level of activity remained more or less stable [31].

Attitudes to sport and the socio-demographic factors that impact on physical activity habits and fitness in adults are complex [12]. Wendell et al. found that experiences that related to participation in physical activity during childhood and adolescence may positively influence physical activity during adulthood. Additionally, researchers have identified that childhood is usually considered to be the best age for socialization into physical activity [32-33]. Similarly, Telama et al. reported that persistent participation in sport as children increased the probability of a higher level of physical activity later in life [34]. Alricsson et al. highlighted that 26 % of high school students in the north of Sweden participated in sport on a regular basis and there were no gender differences identified [35]. In 16 to 18 year old Finnish youths, Aarnio et al. found that those who participated in organised sports were more likely to be fit than those who did not. The Finnish study also reported that 24 to 28 % of the girls and 32 to 36 % of the boys were extremely physically active (4-5 times a week) [33]. This is somewhat less than in the Norwegian and Australian studies (unpublished data) but similar to a Swedish study by Alricsson et al. [35]. This could indicate that the Norwegian and Australian students have reported physical activity when they have performed non organised activity such as when they had probably walked or went by bike to school. Furthermore, Alricsson et al. [35] and unpublished data from Norway and Australia found as have other researchers [16, 31, 36] that a higher number of females participated in physical activities at a lower level of effort (one to three times per week or more) than males, and males participated in activities at a higher level of effort (one to three times or more weekly) than females. This may suggest that males were more likely to take part in competitive sports whereas females were more likely to be involved in recreation sports [35, unpublished data from Norway and Australia]

Allender et al. found that fun, enjoyment and social support were more often the predictors of participation and non-participation in sports than perceived health benefits for teenage girls. Furthermore, a dialectic approach emerged between girls wanting to be physically active and at the same time feminine [3]. Therefore, conflict between sport participation and the ideology of femininity may be reasons for low participation of physical activity in females [38]. Another dimension to physical activity participation of females is a perceived lack of competence and feelings of alienation from being unable to conform to a desired physique.

Similarly, gender-specific motivational factors exist for middle school youths; boys are more attracted to the competitive aspects of sports whereas girls are more motivated by the social opportunities that sports provide [36].

Pfeiffer et al. found that girls who played sports for a higher number of years were more active than non-participants, suggesting that adolescent girls who participated in sports in the eighth, ninth, and twelfth grades have an increased likelihood of being vigorously active in the twelfth grade. Also, maintaining participation to include or surpass a three-year period contributed to a consistent physical activity pattern over time [37].

One of the most important barriers to increased physical activity of youths and especially young women is the recent reduction in physical education programs in schools. This trend might well be reversed if studies demonstrate that physical activity improves classroom behaviour and performance [39]. A committee report that explored physical activity recommendations identified the significance of providing access and resource lists for communities and have highlighted the need for further action. Furthermore, Pate et al. showed that a comprehensive school-based intervention can increase regular participation in vigorous physical activity among high-school girls [40] were continued support from family members may reduce the decline in physical activity independent of a girl's self-efficacy and perceived behavioural control. This correlates with the variables used in growth curve analysis in physical activity over time in adolescent girls [41].

Self-Related Health

Earlier studies have indicated that gender is a powerful predictor of self-related health as often males rate their health higher than females [35, 42, Australian and Norway unpublished data]. Congruent with other research, females consistently rated their health lower than males. Furthermore, physical activity and body mass weight also influence adolescent self-related health [42]. Data collected from previous studies, as well as recent data collected in Australia and Norway [43-45] show that males reported significantly better health than females. These results correlated more positively to Alricsson et al. findings [35] than those presented by Brattberg, who studied school children in a younger age group. However, Brattberg studied health from both a psychological and physiological perspective whereas Alricsson studies were more aligned with self reported health only [46]. Furthermore, the Norwegian (unpublished data) indicated that students in vocational programs reported poorer self-related health than those in academic programs. The males reported better self-related health generally than females in both academic and vocational programs. These findings are similar to Westerståhl et al. study which found that the difference between the educational programs (vocational and academic) correlated with physical activity levels and that vocational programs were associated to lower socio-economic status, lower perceived positive influence from parents to be physically active, as well as lower perceived health among the students in vocational programs [30].

A Canadian study showed a positive relationship between poor mental health and the development of low back pain which is consistent with the research findings in adults [47]. Alricsson et al. found a higher number of females with body complaints reported poorer health than those females without any complaints and the females who were suffering from neck and back pain rated their self-related health to be much worser than males with neck and back pain [35]. This result was similar to that reported by Cho et al. [48]. Therefore, psychological health appears to be a contributing factor related to the musculoskeletal symptoms of adolescents [48].

The consistency of results across different studies is impressive, even though the studies differ with regard to their design, population and the way in which self-related health is assessed. There is no clear definition of what constitutes the attributes of self-related health but often the research reveals that global health status measures physical health problems, functional ability as well as social and mental well-being [49].

BMI (Body Mass Index)

As a measure of relative weight, BMI is easy to obtain (weight in kilos divided by height in square metres, kg/m^2). It is an acceptable proxy for thinness and fatness, and has been directly related to health risks and death rates in many populations. BMI shows significant variations during childhood that is the reason why age and gender specific reference standards must be used. In addition, in adolescents, pubertal status should also be evaluated, since puberty leads to an increase in percentage body fat [50-51].

The most common argument is that young people's lack of participation in sport and physical activity is directly equated with a dramatic rise in childhood obesity [21]. Furthermore, adolescent represents a third critical period when overweight can occur and increase the risks of obesity in adulthood. The risk of becoming overweight during adolescence appears to be higher among girls than among boys, perhaps because adolescence in girls is characterized by a relative increase in fatness due to the period when the BMI begins to increase during the adiposity rebound [52]. The prevalence of overweight and at risk for overweight in children and adolescents now exceeds 30 % and these high levels remain a major public health concern [53].

Janssen et al showed in a review article that overweight and obesity prevalence was particularly high in countries located in North America, Great Britain and South-Western Europe. Within most countries physical activity levels were lower and television viewing times were higher in overweight youths compared to normal weight youths. Increasing physical activity participation and decreasing television viewing should be the focus of strategies aimed at preventing and treating overweight and obesity in youth [54].

The data from the Norwegian and Australian studies, as well as studies from other commentators [55-58] have identified that overweight and obese adolescents showed lower sport participation and had a less positive attitude towards physical activity, in particular girls (unpublished data from Norway and Australia). However, no significant differences were noted in the Norwegian and Australian studies regarding prevalence of overweight in relation to self-related health or body complaints. On the contrary, Vingilis et al. showed that physical activity and BMI influenced self-related health [42]. Several other studies show that there is no strong relation between BMI and low back pain [59-61].

In Norwegian high school students the data supported findings from Westerståhl et al. [30] that there was a higher level of overweight students who were in vocational programs (unpublished data). This might relate to the fact that students in vocational programs often come from a lower socio-economic background were the diet habits are more unhealthy [30].

Attending seminars and expert meetings as well as reading peer reviewed articles on the obesity issue, one may have the feeling that experts have already understood the problems that surround the obesity problem and also know what to do. The solution to the problem seems to be more evident in our discussions then it does in practice. In implementing strategies to deal with the obesity issue we ignore the most important determinant of the overweight epidemic and that is exploring the complexity of the issue. Further studies relating to the problem of overweight should investigate the global problem of obesity at a more complex level that encapsulates the dimensions of societal and community influences, the changing food, work and leisure environments, reconsidering the value and limits of economic growth, and examining the view of obesity (i.e. reducing stigma). Collaborative studies could contribute to reducing the incidence and prevalence of childhood overweight. However, reducing inequalities in health and overweight by emotional, social and financial support is a general and indirect measure of health promotion which in today's political and economic climate may fall short of solving the problem. Today, many experts address the obesity problem directly without tackling the deeper organizational, economic and political affairs that influence our societies [62].

Therefore, responses to address the obesity issue should emanate from all levels of society to improve the health and wellbeing of youths. O´dea found in a study of semi-structured depth focus groups interviews with students aged 13-17 that the identified barriers included a preference for sedentary indoor activities such as television viewing or computer activities, lack of energy and motivation, time constraints, and social factors [63]. Recommended strategies for addressing these barriers included support from parents and school staff, improved planning, and time management, strategies or programs to improve self-motivation, education of the benefits of increased physical activity, and restructuring of the physical environment to be more conducive to a greater choice of physical activities [63]. These factors should be considered when developing physical programs or initiatives that address the overweight and obesity in young women.

Body Complaints

Musculoskeletal symptoms can present early in school-age and it has been suggested that these early symptoms might be the start of a lifelong course of musculoskeletal complaints [49]. The prevalence of the various definitions of low back pain increased greatly in the early teen years, earlier for girls than for boys. By the ages of 18 years for girls and 20 years for boys, more than 50 % had experienced at least one low back pain episode. There is a general tendency for more young women to report low back pain than young men [64]. Sixty-five percent of the female sample in Alricsson et al. study reported that they had experienced body complaints during the last three months, results that are very similar to the Norwegian and Australian results, 73 % and 66 % respectively (unpublished data). Furthermore, Alricsson et al. showed that there were a significantly higher number of females than males who reported complaints with the most common body parts for complaints being the back, knees and neck; the same as in the Norwegian and Australian study [35, Norway and Australia unpublished data]. Similarly, Smedbråten et al. showed that about 50 % of 15 year olds reported body complaints and that knee and back pain were the most frequent areas reported [65]. Females reported more neck and back pain than males [65-66]. These findings are also consistent with findings in the adult population [67-68]. Additionally, research that discusses both female and male back problems from the early age of 16 years indicated that females and girls complained more than boys [32, 61, 69]. There is a variety of reports about back pain in youths. Earlier epidemiological studies in general populations focusing on the age group of 16 to 20 years have shown a history of back pain in 20 to 66 % of individuals and girls reported low back pain more frequently than did boys [35, 46, 69-72]. Therefore, it is important to consider that musculoskeletal symptoms in childhood, particularly if they are frequent, may have important consequences for chronic pain in adulthood [67, 68].

Conclusion

A large number of students reported a high level of symptoms and the reporting of most symptoms increased with age. Girls reported more symptoms than boys and the gender differences also increased with age, more so for girls than boys. These findings indicate that students reported a higher level of subjective health complaints already at an early age and that these findings of health complaints are at two dimensions that differ qualitatively, which suggests that these dimensions may have different etiologies and require differentiated interventions [73].

Introducing a physical dimension to travelling to school for example, walking or cycling could provide an opportunity for increased daily physical activity. Parental support and social support from friends are important for young women, especially in terms of trying out new activities. Furthermore, schools should provide opportunities for young women to participate in a wider range of indoor and leisure activities such as dancing, gymnastics, and aerobics etc. to increase their physical activity and improve their health as numerous studies have shown a positive correlation that young girls participate more frequently in non-competitive organised sports and leisure-activities then young men.

References

[1] Sundblad G, Saartok T, Engström L-M, Renström P. Injuries during physical activity in school children. *Scand. J. Med. Sci. Sports.* 2005; 15:313-23.

[2] Kohl HW, Fulton JE, Caspersen CJ. Assessment of physical activity among children and adolescents: a review and synthesis. *Prev. Med.* 2000; 31:S54-S76.

[3] Allender S, Cowburn G, Foster C. Understanding participation in sport and physical activity among children and adults: a review of qualitative studies. *Health Educ. Res.* 2006; 21:826-35.

[4] Paffenbarger RS, Blair SN, Lee IM. A history of physical activity, cardiovascular health and longevity: the scientific contributions of Jeremy N Morris. *Int. J. pidemiol.* 001; 30:1184-92.

[5] U.S Department of Health and Human Services. *Physical activity and health: a report of the Surgeon General.* Atlanta, (GA): Centers for Disease Control and Prevention, National Center for Chronic Disease Prevention and Health Promotion, 1996.

[6] Hardman AE. Physical activity and health: current issues and research needs. *Int. J. Epidemiol.* 2001; 30:1193-7.

[7] Anderson JJ. The important role of physical activity in skeletal development: how exercise may counter low calcium intake. *Am. J. Clin. Nutr.* 2000; 71:1384-6.

[8] Duppe H, Gardsell P, Johnell O et al. Bone mineral density, muscle strength and physical activity: a population based study of 332 students aged 15-42 years. *Acta Orthop. Scand.* 1997; 68:97-103.

[9] Cameron AJ, Wellborn TA, Zimmet PZ, Dunstan DW, Owen N, Salmon J, Dalton M, Damien J, Shaw JE. Overweight and obesity in Australia: the 1999-2000 Australian diabetes, Obesity and Lifestyle Study. *Med. J. Australia.* 2003; 178(9):427-32.

[10] Pate RR, Pratt M, Blair SN, Haskell WL, Macera CA, Bouchard C, et al. Physical activity and public health. A recommendation from the Centers for Disease Control and Prevention and the American College of Sports Medicine. *JAMA.* 1995; 273:402-7.

[11] Bertelloni S, Ruggeri S, Baroncelli GI. Effects of sports training in adolescence on growth, puberty and bone health. *Gynecol. Endocrinol.* 2006; 22(11):605-12.

[12] Barnekow-Bergkvist M, Hedberg G, Janlert U, Jansson E. Prediction of physical fitness and physical activity level in adulthood by physical performance and physical activity in adolescence – An 18-year follow–up study. *Scand. J. Med. Sci. Sports.* 1998; 8:299-308.

[13] Armstrong N, Welsman JR. The physical activity patterns of European youth with reference to methods of assessment. *Sport Med.* 2006; 36(12):1067-86.

[14] Raustorp A, Pangrazi RP, Ståhle A. Physical activity level and body mass index among schoolchildren in south-eastern Sweden. *Acta Paediatr.* 2004; 93:400-4.

[15] Tudor-Locke C, Pangrazi RP, Corbin CB, Rutherford WJ, Vincent SD, Raustorp A, Tomson LM, Cuddihy TF. BMI-referenced standards for recommended pedometer determined steps/day in children. *Prev. Med.* 2004; 38:857-64.

[16] Sallis JF. Epidemiology of physical activity and fitness in children and adolescents. *Food Sci. Nutr.* 1993; 33:403-8.

[17] Taylor WC, Blair SN, Cummings CC, Wun CC, Malina RM. Childhood and adolescent physical activity patterns and adult physical activity. *Med. Sci. Sports Exerc.* 1999; 31(1):118-23.

[18] Tammelin T, Nayha S, Hills AP, Jarvelin MR. Adolescent participation in sports and adult physical activity. *Am. J. Prev. Med.* 2003; 24(1):22-8.

[19] Dietz WH. Health consequences of obesity in youth: Childhood predictors of adult disease. *Pediatrics.* 1998; 101:518-25.

[20] Hill JO. Trowbridge FL. Childhood obesity: Future directions and research priorities. *Pediatrics.* 1998; 101:570-4.

[21] Brooks F, Magnusson J. Physical activity as leisure: The meaning of physical activity for the health and well-being of adolescent women. *Health Care Women Int.* 2007; (1):69-87.

[22] Caspersen CJ, Powell KE, Christenson GM. Physical activity, exercise, and physical fitness: definitions and distinctions for health-related research. *Public Health Rep.* 1985; 100:126-31.

[23] Pfeiffer KA b), Schmitz KH, McMurray RG, Treuth MS, Murray DM, Pate RR. Physical activities in adolescent girls variability in energy expenditure. *Am. J. Prev. Med.* 2006; 31(4): 328-31.

[24] Raustorp A, Ståhle A, Gudasic H, et al. Physical activity and self-perception in school children assessed with the children and youth-perception profile. *Scand. J. Med. Sci. Sports.* 2005; 15:126-34.

[25] Vincent SD, Pangrazi RP, Raustorp A, et al. Activity levels and body mass index of children in the United states, Sweden and Australia. *Med. Sci. Sport Exerc.* 2003:1367-73.

[26] Sallis JF, Patrick K. Physical activity guidelines for adolescents: consensus statement. *Pediatr. Exerc. Sci.* 1994; 6:302-14.

[27] National Public Health Partnership. *Monitoring and Surveillance of Physical Activity of Children and Young People:* Report of a National Consensus Workshop December 2005. Melbourne NPIIP;2006.

[28] Klasson-Heggebo L, Anderssen SA. Gender and age differences in relation to the recommendations of physical activity among Norwegian children and youth. *Scand. J. Med. Sci. Sports.* 2003; 13:293-8.

[29] Sjolie AN. Associations between activities and low back pain in adolescents. *Scand. J. Med. Sci. Sports.* 2004; 14:352-9.

[30] Westerståhl M, Barnekow-Bergkvist M, Jansson E. Low physical activity among adolescents in practical education. *Scand. J. Med. Sci. Sports.* 2005; 15:287-97.

[31] Mechelen WV, Twisk JWR, Post GB et al. Physical activity of young people: the Amsterdam longitudinal growth and health study. *Med. Sci. Sports Exerc.* 2000;32(9):1610-6.

[32] Wendell CT, Blair SN, Cummings SS, et al. Childhood and adolescent physical activity patterns and adult physical activity. *Med. Sci. Sports Exerc.* 1999; 31:118-23.

[33] Aarnio M,Winter T, Peltonen J, Kujala UM, Kaprio J. Stability of leisure-time physical activity during adolescence. A longitudinal study among 16-, 17- and 18-years-old Finnish youth. *Scand. J. Med. Sci. Sports.* 2002; 12:179-85.

[34] Telama R. Yang X, Laakso L, Viikari J. Physical activity in childhood and adolescence as predictor of physical activity in young adulthood. *Am. J. Prev. Med.* 1997; 13:317-32.

[35] Alricsson M, Landstad BJ, Romild U, Werner S. Self-related health, physical activity and complaints in Swedish high school students. *Scientific World Journal.* 2006; 6: 816-26.

[36] Sirard JR, Pfeiffer KA, Pate RR. Motivational factors associated with sports program participation in middle school students. *J. Adolesc. Health.* 2006; (38): 696-703.

[37] Pfeiffer KA a), Dowda M, Dishman RK, McIver KL, Sirard JR, Ward DS, Pate RR. Sport participation and physical activity in adolescent females across a four-year period. *J. Adolesc. Health.* 2006; 39(4):523-9.

[38] Asci FH, Tuzun M, Koca C. An examination of eating attitudes and physical activity levels of Turkish university students with regard to self-presentational concern. *Eat. Behav.* 2006; 7(4):362-7.

[39] Dietz WH. Physical activity recommendations: where do we go from here? *J. Pediatr.* 2005; 146:719-20.

[40] Pate RR, Ward DS, Saunders RP, Felton G, Dishman RK, Dowda M. Promotion of physical activity among high-school girls: a randomized controlled trial. *Am. J. Public Health.* 2005; 95:1582-7.

[41] Dowda M, Dishman RK, Pfeiffer KA, Pate RR. Family support for physical activity in girls from 8th to 12th grade in South Carolina. *Prev. Med.* 2007; 44:153-9.

[42] Vingilis ER, Wade TJ, Seeley JS. Predictors of Adolescent Self-rated Health. Canadian *Journal of Public Health.* 2002; 93(3):193-7.

[43] Wade TJ, Vingilis E. The Development of self-related health during adolescence: an exploration of inter- and intracohort effects. *Can. J. Public Health.* 1999; 90(2):90-4.

[44] Krause NM, Jay GM. What do global self-rated health items measure. *Med. Care.* 1994; 32(9):930-42.

[45] Vingilis E, Wade TJ, Adlaf EM. What factors predict student self-related physical health? *J. Adolesc.* 1998; 21(1):83-97.

[46] Brattberg G. The incidence of back pain and headache among Swedish school children. *Qual. Life Res.* 1994; 3:27-31.

[47] Ehrmann Feldman D, Shrier I, Rossignol M, Abenhaim L. Risk factors for the development of low back pain in adolescence. *Am. J. Epidemiol.* 2001; 154:30-6.

[48] Cho CY C, Hwang IS, Chen CC. The association between psychological distress and musculoskeletal symptoms experienced by Chinese high school students. *J. Orthop. Sports Phys. Ther.* 2003; 33:344-53.

[49] Undén AL, Elofsson S. Health from the patient's point of view. How does it relate to the physician's judgement? *Family Practice.* 2001; 18:174-80.

[50] Barba C, Cavalli-Sforza T, Cutter J, Darnton-Hill I. Appropriate body-mass index for Asian populations and its implications for policy and intervention strategies. *Lancet.* 2004; 363: 157-63.

[51] Flodmark CE, Lissau I, Pietrobelli A. Child and adolescent obesity: Why we need to fight! *Acta Paediatr.* 2005; 94(448):4-7.

[52] Dietz WH. Overweight in childhood and adolescence. *N. Engl. J. Med.* 2004; 26:350(9):855-7.

[53] Hedley AA, Ogden CL, Johnson CL, Carroll MD, Curtin LR, Flegal KM. Prevalence of overweight and obesity among U.S. children, adolescents, and adults, 1999-2002. *JAMA.* 2004; 291(23):2847-50.

[54] Janssen I, Katzmarzyk PT, Boyce WF, Vereecken C, Mulvihill C, Roberts C, Currie C, Pickett W. Comparison of overweight and obesity prevalence in school-aged youth from 34 countries and their relationships with physical activity and dietary patterns. *Obes. Rev.* 2005; 6:123-32.

[55] Smith BJ, Phongsavan P, Havea D, Halavatau V, Chey T. Body mass index, physical activity and dietary behaviours among adolescents in the kingdom of Tonga. *Public Health Nutr.* 2007; 10(2):137-44.

[56] Yang X, Telama R, Viikari J, Raitakari OT. Risk of obesity in relation to physical activity tracking from youth to adulthood. *Int. J. Obes.* 2007; 31(3):521-7.

[57] Deforche BI, De Bourdeaudhuij IM, Tanghe AP. Attitude toward physical activity in normal-weight, overweight and obese adolescents. *J. Adolesc. Health.* 2006; 38:560-8.

[58] Zabinski MF, Saelens BE, Stein RI, Hayden-Wade HA, Wilfley DE. Overweight children's barriers to and support for physical activity. *Obes. Res.* 2003; 11(2):238-46.

[59] Deyo RA, Bass JE. Lifestyle and low back pain: the influence of smoking and obesity. *Spine.* 1989;14:501-6.
[60] Nachemson AL, Jonsson E. *Neck and back pain.* Philadephia, PA: Lippincott Williams and Wilkins; 2000.
[61] Kovacs FM, Gestoso M, Gil del Real MT, Lopez J, Mufraggi N, Mendez JI. Risk factors for non-specific low back pain in schoolchildren and their parents: a population based study. *Pain.* 2003; 103(3):259-68.
[62] Müller MJ, Danielzik S. Childhood overweight: is there need for a new societal approach to the obesity epidemic? *Obes. Rev.* 2007; 8 87-90.
[63] O'Dea JA. Why do kids eat healthful food? Perceived benefits of and barriers to healthful eating and physical activity among children and adolescents. *J. AM. Diet Assoc.* 2003; 103:497-501.
[64] Leboeuf-Yde C, Kyvik KO. At what age does low back pain become a common problem? A study of 29,424 individuals aged 12-41 years. *Spine.* 1998; 15; 23(2):228-34.
[65] Smedbråten BK, Natvig B, Rutle O. Self-reported bodily pain in schoolchildren. *Scand. J. Rheumatol.* 1998; 27:273-6.
[66] Brun Sundblad GM, Saartok T, Engström LM. Prevalence and co-occurrence of self-rated pain and perceived health in school-children: Age and gender differences. *Eur. J. Pain.* 2007; 11(2):171-80.
[67] Brattberg G. Do pain problems in young school children persist into early adulthood? A 13-year follow up. *Eur. J. Pain.* 2004; 8:187-99.
[68] Watson KD, Papageorgiou AC, Jones GT, Taylor S, Symmons DPM, Silman AJ, Macfarlane GJ. Low back pain in schoolchildren: occurrence and characteristics. *Pain.* 2002; 97(1-2):87-92.
[69] Borge AIH, Nordhagen R. Recurrent pain symptoms in children and parents. *Acta Paediatr.* 2000; 89:1479-83.
[70] Kujala UM, Taimela S, Viljanen T. Leisure physical activity and various pain symptoms among adolescents. *Br. J. Sports Med.* 1999; 33:325-8.
[71] Balagué F, Dutoit G, Waldburger M. Low back pain in schoolchildren. *Scand. J. Rehabil. Med.* 1988; 20:175-9.
[72] Balagué F, Nordin M, Skovron ML. Non-specific low-back pain among schoolchildren: A field survey with analysis of some associated factors. *J. Spinal. Disord.* 1994; 7(5):374-9.
[73] Haugland S. Wold B. Stevenson J, Aaroe LE, Woynarowska B. Subjective health complaints in adolescence. *Eur. J. Public Health.* 2001; 11:4-10.

About the Authors

Marie Alricsson, PhD, RPT, is a physiotherapist and graduated at the Karolinska Institutet, Stockholm. She has a PhD in sports medicine from the Karolinska Institutet, Stockholm and has done her post doctoral studies in Griffith University, Queensland, Australia. Her research and publications are in the area of public health, prevention, sports medicine and rehabilitation. She is working as a researcher and a senior lecturer in rehabilitation science at the Mid Sweden University, Department of Health Sciences, SE- 831 25 Östersund, Sweden. E-mail: marie.alricsson@miun.se

Debra Domalewski's degree studies are in the Human Services Discipline, majoring in Rehabilitation Counselling at Griffith University, Brisbane, Australia. Her research interests and publications are in the area of community rehabilitation education and competencies, research partnerships, case management and population health. She is working as a researcher at the Disability and Rehabilitation Research Unit, Research Centre for Clinical Innovation, Griffith University, Logan Campus , Meadowbrook. QLD. Australia. 4131. E-mail: d.domalewski@griffith.edu.au.

In: Exercise and Women's Health
Editor: Laura A. Charlington, pp. 157-167
ISBN: 978-1-60456-013-8

Chapter 8

HIV/AIDS, EXERCISE AND WOMEN'S HEALTH RESEARCH

Julie Hard*[*1], *Stephanie A. Nixon*[*2], *Kelly O'Brien*[*3], *Anne-Marie Tynan*[*4] and *Richard H. Glazier*[*5]

[1] Inner City Health Programme, St. Michael's Hospital, 30 Bond Street, 14th Floor, Toronto, Ontario, M5V 1W8, Canada

[2] Department of Physical Therapy, Faculty of Medicine, 160-500 University Avenue, Toronto, Ontario, M5G 1V7, Canada, and Health Economics and HIV/AIDS Research Division (HEARD), University of KwaZulu-Natal, Westville Campus, J-Block, Durban, South Africa

[3] Department of Physical Therapy, Faculty of Medicine, 160-500 University Avenue, Toronto, Ontario, M5G 1V7, Canada

[4] Centre for Research on Inner City Health, St. Michael's Hospital, 70 Richmond Street, 4th Floor, Toronto, Ontario, M5C 1N8, Canada

[5] Institute for Clinical Evaluative Sciences, Centre for Research on Inner City Health at St. Michael's Hospital, and Family and Community Medicine, University of Toronto and St. Michael's Hospital, G1-06, 2075 Bayview Avenue, Toronto, Ontario, M4N 3M5, Canada

ABSTRACT

The purpose of this chapter is to present an overview of evidence on the effects of exercise in women living with HIV in order to identify directions for future research. To this end, we present a synthesis of research on a variety of HIV and exercise outcomes, including immunological, virological, cardiopulmonary, musculoskeletal, body composition and psychological effects, with reflection on the relevance of these findings

* hardj@smh.toronto.on.ca
* stephanie.nixon@utoronto.ca
* kelly.obrien@utoronto.ca
* tynanma@smh.toronto.on.ca
* rick.glazier@ices.on.ca

for women. We conclude that, given (a) the significance of exercise as a therapeutic strategy for people living with HIV, (b) the feminization of the HIV pandemic, (c) the unique considerations related to gender and exercise, and (d) the paucity of evidence on the effects of exercise in women living with HIV, further research is urgently needed to explore the safety and effectiveness of aerobic and progressive resistive exercise in women living with HIV. Such research should take into account methodological lessons learned from existing studies, which have been conducted primarily with male adults living with HIV. Future research should also take into account unique considerations pertaining to women living with HIV, including metabolic and hormonal features, as well as the different social demands, circumstances and context of women's lives.

INTRODUCTION

Consider these scenarios. A 39-year-old Canadian woman has been HIV-positive for five years. She started highly active antiretroviral therapy (HAART) three years ago and has watched her immune status steadily improve. However, she has been daunted by changes to the appearance of her body associated with lipodystrophy syndrome. She has a noticeable thickening of fat around her abdomen, and her arms and legs appear to be wasting away. She is wondering whether a weight-training programme will help her to reverse these changes – and whether it will be safe given her HIV-positive status.

On the other side of the world, a 25-year-old South African mother of four has been newly diagnosed with HIV. HAART is not yet indicated in the early stage of her disease. She enjoys a vigorous walk with friends each morning. She wonders whether she ought to increase this aerobic exercise in order to strengthen her body against future HIV-related illnesses, or whether she should stop pushing her body like this now that she is HIV-positive.

Although these women come from different parts of the world, they share concerns about the impact of exercise on their health and well-being. Women now comprise approximately 50% of the 38 million people estimated to be living with HIV worldwide. In sub-Saharan Africa, women represent an estimated 59% of adults living with HIV.[1] In developed countries like Canada, the proportion of women living with HIV is lower, but the incidence of HIV among women is on the rise in many environments. As such, research on therapeutic strategies for women is more important than ever before.

Exercise is one strategy that has been used by people living with HIV in an effort to prevent future complications, minimize existing disablement, reduce side effects from HAART and achieve psychological benefits. However, the bulk of research on the effects of exercise in people living with HIV has focused on the experience of men.

A recent Cochrane Collaboration systematic review of the effects of progressive resistive exercise in adults living with HIV revealed potential benefits for body weight and composition with exercise compared with no exercise.[2] However, only one of the seven randomized controlled trials in the review involved women,[3] resulting in women accounting for only 15% of the participants in the overall review.

A second systematic review examined the effects of aerobic exercise or a combination of aerobic and progressive resistive exercise in adults living with HIV. This review revealed potential improvements in selected outcomes of cardiopulmonary status and psychological status among exercisers compared to non-exercisers. However, only four of the eleven randomized controlled trials reviewed included women as participants.[4] Of these studies, women represented less than 15% of the total number of participants. Furthermore, results from the reviewed studies were not reported by gender and, therefore, no analysis could be performed regarding the impact that exercise may have on women versus men.

Although these reviews included only randomized controlled trials, research on exercise and HIV using other study designs provides little additional insight on effects for women. As a result, guidance for exercise prescription in women living with HIV has to be inferred from evidence based on studies predominantly comprised of men.

The purpose of this chapter is to provide an overview of the evidence on the effects of exercise in women living with HIV in order to identify directions for future research. To this end, we present a synthesis of research on a variety of exercise outcomes, including immunological, virological, cardiopulmonary, musculoskeletal, body composition and psychological effects, with reflection on the relevance of these findings for women. We finish by describing future directions for research to address the gaps in current knowledge on the effects of exercise in women living with HIV.

Immunological and Virological Outcomes

Disease progression in HIV/AIDS is commonly monitored through an immunological marker known as CD4 count and a virological marker called viral load. CD4 lymphocytes, which are required for healthy functioning of the immune system, are a primary target of HIV. As the number of CD4 cells declines, individuals are increasingly susceptible to a range of opportunistic infections, malignancies and disease syndromes. Viral load, measured in number of copies of HIV per millilitre of blood, indicates the amount of virus circulating in the blood. As the virus replicates in the body, the measure of HIV viral load increases. The higher the viral load, the more active HIV is in the body.

Several studies have examined the effects of exercise on these immunological and/or virological indicators in people living with HIV. Results from meta-analyses comparing the effects of various types of aerobic exercise interventions (i.e. constant or interval aerobic exercise, moderate or high intensity aerobic exercise, aerobic exercise alone or combined with progressive resistive exercise) when compared to non-exercising controls demonstrated no statistically significant difference in CD4 count for participants in the exercise group when compared to the non-exercising control group.[4] Further meta-analysis also demonstrated no statistical difference in CD4 percentage or change in viral load between exercisers and non-exercisers in aerobic studies.[4]

Similarly, results from a systematic review examining progressive resistive exercise or a combination of progressive resistive and aerobic exercise at least three times per week for four weeks, demonstrated no change in CD4 count or viral load among exercisers compared with non-exercisers.[2] While the majority of studies in these reviews primarily included men, it appears that participation in aerobic exercise, progressive resistive exercise, or a combination of aerobic and progressive resistive exercise at least three times per week for at least four weeks is safe, meaning it does not appear to have negative immunological or virological consequences for adults living with HIV who are medically stable.[2,4]

Recently, a single randomized controlled trial examined the immunological response to aerobic exercise over a longer intervention period with women representing 30% of the participants who completed the trial.[5] In this study, 42 adults (CD4 >250 cells/mm3) with HIV and dyslipidemia receiving HAART, were randomized to either a 12-week program of aerobic exercise combined with a low-lipid diet or a program of stretching and relaxation with a low-lipid diet. Results of the study revealed a decrease in mean CD4 count in the exercise group of 41 cells/mm^3. However, this change was not statistically significant ($p=0.35$), nor was there a significant effect of the intervention on viral load ($p=0.39$). Differences between genders were not reported. Overall, however, the aerobic exercise programme of longer duration for these participants did not appear to negatively impact immune status. In other words, in these studies, exercise appeared to be safe for people living with HIV.

Cardiopulmonary Outcomes

Cardiac abnormalities are commonly associated with HIV infection and can exacerbate symptoms of fatigue and activity intolerance.[6,7] Compared to the general population, adults living with HIV are at an increased risk for coronary heart disease and acute myocardial infarction (MI), which is further increased for those receiving HAART treatment.[8,9,10] Women living with HIV, in particular, have an increased number of cardiovascular risk factors compared to women who are HIV-negative.[11] Moreover, results of a longitudinal cohort study (1996-2004) comparing MI rates between adults with and without HIV revealed that women living with HIV are at an increased risk of experiencing an MI compared to women in the general population, even after adjusting for age, ethnicity, hypertension, dyslipidemia and diabetes (RR = 2.98, 95% CI 2.33 – 3.75; $p<0.0001$).[12]

Studies investigating cardiopulmonary response to exercise in people living with HIV have used a range of exercise prescriptions and outcome measures, which has limited the potential for meta-analysis. However, improvements in maximum oxygen consumption (VO_2max) were reported in three separate meta-analyses that assessed the response of aerobic exercise or aerobic exercise combined with progressive resistive exercise when compared to non-exercising control groups of adults living with HIV.[4]

Improvements in VO_2max of 1.64, 1.53, and 4.30 mL/kg/min were found with continuous or interval aerobic exercise compared with non-exercise (meta-analysis of 4 studies), continuous exercise compared to non-exercise (3 studies), and moderate intensity compared with heavy intensity exercise (2 studies), respectively. Those exercising at heavy-intensity exercise demonstrated a potentially clinically important improvement in cardiopulmonary function beyond those exercising at moderate intensity.[4] The same review revealed a trend towards a decrease in maximum heart rate (HRmax) with aerobic exercise training, although this change was not statistically significant.

In a recent prospective, longitudinal pilot study, 28 women living with HIV and obesity (defined as having a BMI >30 kg/m^2) completed a combined aerobic and progressive resistive exercise programme over 12 weeks.[13] The exercise intervention included moderate intensity treadmill training at 70-80% of estimated maximal heart rate for 30 minutes followed by progressive resistance exercises for seven major muscle groups, three times per week. Cardiopulmonary fitness was assessed as length of time on treadmill and perceived exertion during treadmill activity. Results reported an increase in amount of time sustained on a treadmill from baseline before reaching 85% of maximum heart rate from 8.8 +/- 3.3 to 10.9

+/- 2.4 minutes (36.8% +/- 41.6%, p=.0015) and reported a decrease in perceived exertion from 14.9 +/- 2.1 to 13.7 +/- 1.5 (-7.2% to 14.8%, p=.03). These findings are consistent with improvements seen in fitness levels reported by the general population and demonstrate an overall trend toward improved cardiopulmonary health with aerobic exercise for women living with HIV.

Musculoskeletal Outcomes

Research suggests that progressive resistance exercise can build muscular strength for women living with HIV.[3,13] In one randomized controlled trial comparing the effects of progressive resistance exercise (PRE), PRE combined with whey protein, and whey protein alone, women in both exercise groups experienced significant strength gains.[3] For 14 weeks, the participants performed 3 sets (8-10 repetitions) of ten supervised resistive exercises at 75% of a one-repetition maximum (1-RM). Improvements in strength for target muscle groups at the end of the intervention period ranged from 40.6% to 95.3%, (p<.001) for the PRE alone group. Participants in the PRE combined with whey protein group also demonstrated slight improvements in strength (6.6% - 16.9%, p=.01-.12).

In a prospective, longitudinal study of 28 women living with HIV and obesity, the effects of a program of energy restriction (diet) combined with aerobic and resistance exercises were assessed for a number of health outcomes, including strength.[13] The exercise intervention consisted of a 30-minute aerobic exercise program of moderate intensity (70-80% of HRmax) followed by 10 resistance exercises for 7 major muscle groups. Strength was assessed as changes in 1-RM at the end of the 12-week program. Participants demonstrated a 30% increase in strength from baseline upon completion of the programme (p<.0001).

Although the sample sizes in each of these studies were small, the women living with HIV demonstrated an overall increase in muscular strength with PRE alone, PRE combined with whey protein or PRE combined with aerobic exercise.

Body Composition Outcomes

Body composition changes (both increases and decreases) are common among people living with HIV and are evaluated through direct or indirect measures of muscle, fat, bone and other body tissues. A common cause of body composition changes is HIV-related wasting syndrome, which is defined as the involuntary loss of greater than 10% of baseline body weight in combination with diarrhea, weakness or fever.[14] The role of exercise as a therapeutic intervention is particularly important since the severity of illness associated with HIV-related wasting appears to be related more to changes in body composition (i.e., proportion of fat and muscle), than to changes in weight.[15]

Since the advent of HAART in the mid-1990's, an additional cause of weight or fat mass redistribution is HIV-associated lipodystrophy, a syndrome in which some areas of the body (e.g. abdomen, breasts, upper back) may experience increases in fat deposition while wasting occurs in other areas (e.g. arms, legs, cheeks). This syndrome is also associated with metabolic abnormalities, including insulin resistance, diabetes and hyperlipidemia.

In terms of the role that exercise can play in addressing these body composition changes, one meta-analysis has demonstrated that significant increases in weight (4.24 kg) were achieved in a PRE group compared with non-exercising controls.[2] In a second meta-analysis, statistically significant changes in body composition (increase in arm and thigh girth by 7.91 cm) were achieved among PRE or combined PRE and aerobic exercisers versus non-exercising controls.[2] Given that many of the participants in these studies had been diagnosed with wasting syndrome, increases in weight and body composition were considered favourable outcomes.

In one study involving adults (30% of whom were women) with HIV-related wasting syndrome, a 12-week randomized controlled trial compared PRE three times per week to oral androgen interventions.[16] The PRE group demonstrated a significant increase in mid-thigh cross-sectional muscle area (5% +/- 2% from baseline) as measured by computed tomography (CT) when compared to diet and diet with oral androgen[16]

Improvements were seen in muscle cross-sectional area in another 12-week study of adults (20% women) with HIV-associated lipodystrophy. In this study, combined resistive and aerobic exercise with metformin (an antidiabetic medication that reduces glucose production), resulted in increased mid-thigh cross-sectional area on CT (3 cm^2 [-3, 12; p=0.02]) when compared to metformin alone, which decreased muscle cross-sectional area of the thigh (-7cm^2 [-11,0; p=0.02]).[17]

A third study, which exclusively examined women living with HIV, demonstrated significant increases in body cell mass in a combined resistive and aerobic exercise group (0.74 kg; $p<0.05$) and in a combined whey protein and exercise group (0.61 kg; $p<0.05$).[3] Skeletal muscle was also determined to have significantly increased in the same study for the PRE only group (1.2 kg; $p<0.001$), but not for the combined whey protein and exercise or whey protein only groups.

Increased muscle cross-sectional area, body cell mass and skeletal muscle are believed to have beneficial impacts for combating the effects of wasting diseases, maintaining strength and contributing to overall physical fitness for people with HIV.[16] The existing evidence suggests that exercise may be beneficial for increasing muscle mass and alleviating the effects of wasting syndromes in women living with HIV, although results should be interpreted cautiously given small sample sizes, number of male subjects included in the results and variability in study design methodologies.

Psychological Outcomes

The measurement of psychological responses to exercise is important for women living with HIV, especially due to the high levels of depression reported in this population. In a recent Cochrane Collaboration systematic review, seven of eleven studies examining aerobic exercise evaluated psychological status outcomes in people living with HIV.[4] Due to the heterogeneity in interventions and outcome measures, meta-analysis was limited to two studies, neither of which included women in their final analyses.[18,19]

Although evaluating only male participants, meta-analysis of the depression-dejection subscale from the Profile of Mood States (POMS) outcome measure demonstrated a statistically significant and possible clinically important reduction in depressive symptoms among participants engaged in aerobic exercise three times per week at 60% -80% of HRmax when compared to non-exercisers.[4] Results from individual studies in the review, which included a small percentage of women, reported positive outcomes among participants in aerobic exercise groups when compared to controls in terms of anxiety, depression, mood and life satisfaction and general health, suggesting that aerobic exercise may be beneficial for psychological health in people living with HIV.

Similarly, another systematic review examining PRE for people living with HIV found that three of the seven included studies reporting on psychological status.[2] Of these studies, two found that participants in exercise groups versus control groups reported improvements in health-related quality of life measures, higher positive mood and lower negative mood with exercise intervention.[3,20] The remaining study reported no difference in changes in health-related quality of life measures between groups.[21]

Interpreting Study Results Cautiously

In summary, aerobic exercise, PRE, or a combination of aerobic and PRE exercise appear to be safe and may lead to improvements in maximum oxygen consumption, strength, weight and body composition, and psychological health in adults living with HIV. However, these results are largely based on the experience of male study participants and, thus, implications for women should be made with caution. Furthermore, even the research involving male participants has a number of shortcomings.

First, the overall number of studies in this area is small. Meta-analyses of randomized controlled trials were only able to combine data from two to four studies. Within this small number of studies, the methodological quality of the included studies varied. Participant withdrawal rates were high, which compromises generalizability since the overall findings among those who continued to exercise might not reflect the experience of exercise among all adults living with HIV/AIDS. Additionally, publication bias may have occurred if trials with negative results were suppressed in the published literature, leaving mostly small but positive studies for review.

A further shortcoming is that studies could not achieve participant blinding due to the nature of the intervention of interest, i.e., exercise. This may have led to bias in the results such as the Hawthorne effect whereby participants may perceive greater benefits associated with exercise based on the expectation that the intervention should be linked to positive outcomes. Study reports were vague in their descriptions of the level of assessor blinding. If assessors were not blinded to the allocation of participants to groups, this may have resulted in detection bias whereby assessors that know group allocation may assess participants in the exercise intervention groups differently than participants in the non-exercising control group. This may lead to more positive outcomes in exercisers compared to non-exercisers based on the assessor's perception that exercise should be linked to positive outcomes.

In addition, many of the studies were susceptible to performance bias due to the difference in the level of interaction between the study investigators and participants in the exercise groups compared with the non-exercising control groups. Participants in the exercise groups were followed three times per week resulting in far greater interaction with study investigators compared to the non-exercising control participants. Participants followed more closely by investigators may tend to report more positive subjective outcomes, such as health-related quality of life, compared to participants that had less extensive interaction.

Future Directions for Exercise Research in Women Living with HIV

Given (a) the significance of exercise as a therapeutic strategy for people living with HIV, (b) the feminization of the HIV pandemic, (c) the unique considerations related to gender and exercise, and (d) the paucity of evidence on the effects of exercise in women living with HIV, further research is needed to explore the safety and effectiveness of aerobic and progressive resistive exercise in women living with HIV.

Future research design may include multi-centred randomized trials that compare the effects of aerobic and progressive resistive exercise among women in intervention and control groups, as well as in women versus men, in order to inform exercise prescription guidelines. Such studies should investigate a range of outcomes including virological, immunological, cardiopulmonary, musculoskeletal, body composition and psychological responses to exercise. Furthermore, future study design should learn from the shortcomings of current research in terms of sample sizes, participant retention and assessor blinding.

Future exercise research should take into account unique considerations of women living with HIV in contrast to men. For instance, gender differences in fat redistribution and wasting syndromes point to opportunities for investigating how exercise may influence fat metabolism in women compared to men living with HIV. In the last decade, the prevalence of lipodystrophy syndrome has increased as a result of metabolic complications of HIV and physiological interactions with HAART. In a cross-sectional analysis of 265 adults living with HIV, no significant difference between genders in total weight and fat mass was found using dual energy X-ray absorptiometry.[22] However, women's experiences with body fat alterations may be different than those of men. Women may demonstrate a unique deposition of fat in the breasts and an increase in abdominal adiposity with subcutaneous fat wasting occurring primarily in the legs.[23,24]

Such alterations in fat distribution can have an impact not only on cardiovascular health, since visceral fat increases risk of cardiovascular complications, but also on psychological well-being and perceptions of body image. Changes in body composition that may be perceived as identifying markers of HIV-positive status may also have serious implications for women for whom disclosure of HIV-seropositivity holds the potential to put them at risk of extreme stigmatization and violence.[25]

Hormonal differences between genders also signal the need for exercise intervention studies to focus specifically on women. Studies in men have demonstrated that lower testosterone levels correlate with a loss of lean body and muscle mass, decreased CD4 cell counts and an increased incidence of opportunistic infections.[26] Women with lower baseline levels of testosterone also have shown declining levels of testosterone, particularly for those experiencing wasting syndromes associated with HIV.[27]

Additional research is required to explore the feasibility of exercise programmes and participant adherence in the context of the social roles that women often maintain within their families and communities. Adherence to exercise programmes for people living with HIV can depend on an individual's physical health status at a given time.[28] For women, adherence to exercise programmes may also be influenced by family commitments and care-giving roles that have not been reported in studies on men. In one study, seven out of the eleven participants who dropped out of the aerobic exercise intervention programme were females citing lack of interest, time, economic or family problems as the reason for discontinuing participation.[5] Another study reported that at the onset of their clinical trial, 23 of the 66 women eligible for participation were disqualified based on family constraints; two participants later dropped out of the study for the same reason.[3] Thus, the role of women as caregivers needs to be considered when determining the nature and practicality of exercise interventions. For instance, interventions could increase the flexibility of exercise times to meet busy schedules, build in parenting and other tasks as part of exercise prescription, or include onsite child-care as part of the exercise programme.

A final consideration for future research involves the appropriateness of different exercise interventions for women in different parts of the world. The era of HIV intervention research based solely on the needs of people living with HIV in developed countries is over. All of the studies reviewed in this article have been conducted in developed country settings. It is crucial that future research efforts seek to understand how exercise and its benefits can best be pursued in different regional and cultural contexts. The Canadian and South African women introduced at the start of this chapter share may commonalities. However, they will also likely differ in terms of the meanings they attach to exercise and the social, political and economic environments in which they live. These same contrasts can also be found among women *within* Canada and *within* South Africa. As such, future research should endeavour to take into account not only the efficacy of exercise in women living with HIV, but also the effectiveness of exercise programmes in the context of their unique lives and circumstances.

REFERENCES

[1] Joint United Nations Programme on HIV/AIDS (UNAIDS). *2006 Report on the Global AIDS Epidemic*. Geneva, Switzerland: UNAIDS. July 2006.

[2] O'Brien, K; Nixon, S; Glazier, RH; Tynan, AM. Progressive resistive exercise interventions for adults living with HIV/AIDS. *The Cochrane Database of Systematic Reviews,* 2004, Issue 4. Art. No.: CD004248.pub2. DOI: 10.1002/14651858. CD004248.pub2.

[3] Agin, D; Gallager, D; Wang J; Heymsfield, SB; et al. Effects of whey protein and resistance exercis on body cell mass, muscle strength, and quality of life in women with HIV. *AIDS,* 2001 15:2431-2440.

[4] O'Brien, K; Nixon, S; Tynan, AM; Glazier, RH. Aerobic exercise interventions for people living with HIV/AIDS: Implications for practice, education, and research. *Physiother. Can,* 2006;58:114-129.

[5] Terry, L; Sprinz, E; Stein, R; et al. Exercise training in HIV-1-infected individuals with dyslipidemia and lipodystropy. *Med. Sci. Sports Exerc,* 2006;38(3):411-417.

[6] Rerkpattanapipat, P; Wongpraparut, N; Jocobs, LE; Kotler, MN. Cardiac manifestations of acquired immunodeficiency syndrome. *Arch. Intern. Med,* 2000;160:602-608.

[7] Yunis, NA; Stone, VE. Cardiac manifestations of HIV/AIDS: a review of disease spectrum and clinical management. *J. Acquir. Immune Defic. Syndr. Hum. Retrovirol,* 1998;18:145-154.

[8] Klein, D; Hurley, LB; Quesenberry, Jr. CP; Sidney, S. Do protease inhibitors increase the risk for coronary heart disease in patients with HIV-1 infection? *J. Acquir. Immune Defic. Syndr,* 2002;30:471-477.

[9] Obel, N; Thomsen, HF; Kronborg, G; Larsen, CS; et al. Ischemic heart disease in HIV-infected and HIV uninfected individuals: a population based cohort study. *Clin. Infect. Dis,* 2007;44(12):1625-1631.

[10] Mary-Krause, M; Cotte, L; Simon, A; Partisani, M; et al. Increased risk of myocardial infarction with duration of protease inhibitor therapy in HIV infected men. *AIDS,* 2003;17:2479-2486.

[11] Dolan, S; Hadigan, C; Killilea, K; Sullivan, M; et al. Increased cardiovascular diseases risk indices in HIV infected women. *J. Acquir. Immune Syndr,* 2005;39:44-54.

[12] Triant, VA; Lee, H; Hadigan, C; Grinspoon, SK. Increased acute myocardial infarction rates and cardiovascular risk factors among patients with HIV disease. *J. Clin. Endocrinol. Metab,* 2007;92(7):2506-2512.

[13] Engelson, ES; Agin, D; Kenya, S; Werber-Zion, G; et al. Body composition and metabolic effects of a diet and exercise weight loss regimen on obese, HIV-infected women. *Metabolism,* 2006;55:1327-1336.

[14] Centers for Disease Control and Prevention. Revision of the CDC surveillance case definition for acquired immunodeficiency syndrome. *MMWR Morb. Mortal. Wkly. Rep.* 36(2S):3S-15S, 1987.

[15] Dudgeon, WD; Phillips, KD; Bopp, CM; Hand GA. Physiological and psychological effects of exercise interventions in HIV disease. *AIDS Patient Care STDS,* 2004;18:81-98.

[16] Shevitz, AH; Wilson, IB; McDermott, AY; Spiegelman, D; et al. A comparison of the clinical and cost-effectiveness of 3 intervention strategies for AIDS wasting. *J. Acquir. Immine Defic. Syndr,* 2005;38(4):399-406.

[17] Driscoll, SD; Meininger GE; Ljungquist, K; Hadigan, C; et al. Differential effects of metformin and exercise on muscle adiposity and metabolic indices in human immunodeficiency virus-infected patients. *J. Clin. Endocrinol. Metab,* 2004;89(5)2171-2178.

[18] LaPierre, AR; Antoni, H; Schneiderman, N; Ironson, G; et al. Exercise intervention attenuates emotional distress and natural killer cell decrements following notification of positive serologic status for HIV-1. *Biofeedback Self Regul,* 1990;15:229-242.

[19] Smith, BA; Neidig, JL; Nickel, JT; Mitchell, GL; et al. Aerobic exercise: effects on parameters related to fatigue, dyspnea, weight and body compostion in HIV -infected adults. *AIDS,* 2001;15:693-701.

[20] Lox, CL; McAuley, E; Tucker RS. Exercise as an intervention for enhancing subjective well-being in an HIV-1 population. *J. Sprot Exerc. Psychol,* 1995;17:345-362.

[21] Bhasin, S; Storer, TW; Javanbakht, M; Berman, N; et al. Testosterone replacement and resistance exercise in HIV-infected men with weight loss and low testosterone levels. *JAMA,* 2000;283(6):763-770.

[22] McDermott, AY; Shevitz, A; Knox, T; Roubenoff, R; et al. Effects of highly active antiretroviral therapy on fat, lean, and bone mass in HIV-seropositive men and women. *Am. J. Clin. Nutr,* 2001;74:679-86.

[23] Ridolfo, AL; Gervasoni, C; Bini, T; Galli, M. Body habitus alterations in HIV infected women treated with combined anti-retroviral therapy. *AIDS Patient Care and STDS,* 2000;14(11):595-601.

[24] Gervasoni, C; Ridolfo, AL; Trifiro, G; Trabattoni, D; et al. Redistribution of body fat in HIV infected women undergoing combined antiretroviral therapy. *AIDS,* 1999;13:465-47.

[25] Gray, J. The difficulties of women living with HIV infection. *J. Psychosoc. Nurs. Ment. Health Serv,* 1999;37:39-45.

[26] Kopicko, JJ; Momodu, I; Adedokun, A; Hoffman, M; et al. Characteristics of HIV infected men with low serum testosterone levels. *Int. J. STD AIDS,* 1999;10:817-820.

[27] Grinspoon, S; Corocoran, C; Miller, K; Biller BMK; et al. Body composition and endocrine function in women with acquired immunodeficiency syndrome wasting. *J. Clin. Endocrinol. Metab,* 1997;82:1332-1337.

[28] Pavone, RM; Burnett, KF; LaPerriere, A; Perna, FM. Social cognitive and physical health determinants of exercise adherence for HIV-1 seropositive, early symptomatic men and women. *Intl. J. of Behav. Med,* 1998:5(3);245-258.

INDEX

B

C

D

E

I

J

K

L

M

N

O

P

Q

R

S

T

U

V

W

Y